Salvaged Souls

By Keith Bennett

Note from the Author:

This is a work of fiction. Any resemblance to actual persons living or dead or references to locations, persons, events or locations is purely coincidental. The characters, circumstances and events are imaginative and not intended to reflect real events.

Coming Soon:

- Street Justice

Join Keith on FB at http://www.facebook.com/Keith.Bennett

Chapter 1

Be merciful unto me O God, be merciful unto me. For my soul trusteth in thee. Yea, in the shadow of thy wings will I make my refuge, until these calamites be over past. Psalms 57:1

This is a prayer I prayed every morning as soon as my feet hit the floor. I once lived the life of a condemned man in a world full of sin until my Lord came and salvaged my soul. Hello brothers and sisters, my name is Victor Wilson and this is my testimony.

My story goes back to my 21st birthday in 1991. I was going out with a couple friends to celebrate.

"Yo, Victor, do you want some of this, man?" James Thomas, my best friend since junior high school asked me.

James was one of the local big time drug dealers who ran most of Chattanooga's coke business. He influenced me to take my first sniff of cocaine.

"Yeah, James, I'll take a sniff of that sunshine." I said coming out the bathroom looking at the beautiful, young lady James brought for me to celebrate my birthday with.

Her name was Tiffany. She was drop dead gorgeous. Tiffany was 22 years old, stood about 5'10", with caramel skin, a nice body, a short hairstyle, and brown contacts in her eyes. She was doing coke with James, his girlfriend and me. We did a couple lines before we left my apartment.

We arrived at the club at around 10. Everyone screamed out, "Happy birthday, Vic," as I walked through the door. I was surprised to see so many people at my birthday party. James paid for everything including the invitations. He had all our friends and some of the local jokers that did business with him in attendance. Of course, I didn't mind.

We went up to the VIP section James reserved for us and we started partying. During the night, I drank on Dom and tooted about three grams of powder. Tiffany hung by my side the whole night. Around three in the morning, I decided that I had had enough and it was time to go. Tiffany and I left the party and went back to my place. When we got there, we did about another gram of coke and then made love until the morning came.

"What time is it, Vic?" Tiffany asked.

"It's 7:30 Tiffany, Why? Do you have somewhere to be?" I asked.

"Naw, Victor, but I have to take my medicine at 8:00," She said.

"What type of medicine are you taking, Tiffany?"

"My birth control and medicine for sickle cell."

"Oh, I didn't know that you had sickle cell."

"Yeah, Victor, but it only gives me problems when I drink a lot of liquor like we did last night. I have to take my medication before it kicks all the way in because if not, I'll be in a lot of pain." She reached into her purse and removed four pill bottles and went into the kitchen to get some water. After she left the room, I went to the bathroom to take the condom off. That's when I realized the condom had busted. I didn't give it much thought because Tiffany said she was on birth control, so I kept it to myself. Why make a big issue over a busted condom and lose the chance of getting some more of that fine loving, I thought. When Tiffany came back to the bedroom, we made love once more then went back to sleep.

Later that day, Tiffany woke, got dressed and left. Leaving me alone trying to get over the hangover from last night. I was making a sandwich when the phone rang.

"Hello?"

"Hey, my man, Vic." James' voice came loudly through the phone and I held it back from my ear. "How did you enjoy last night?" he asked.

"I had a ball, James. But I'm feeling it now. Thanks for everything."

"No problem, Vic. You're my boy, man. What about Tiffany? Did she rock your 21st last night?"

"She was ok, James."

"Ahh, Vic! She had to be more than ok! She's the best money can buy."

"Buy?" I asked.

"Yeah, playa, she's a working girl."

"What, James!" I yelled out. "You set me up with a whore, man?"

"Man, she's straight, Vic. She's one of my playas girls."

"Damn, James! You know I don't get down like that. Those girls be sexing with any and everybody, playa!"

"So what, Vic. I know you didn't hit her raw. Did you?" James asked.

"Naw, James, you know me better than that." However, at the same time, I was thinking about the condom busting and about her having sickle cell. "Man, I hope she was straight, James. I let her give me head without a condom."

"Ahh, Vic, stop trippin' like that, playa. My boy makes his girls go get checked out every six months anyway. I don't think you can catch anything from oral, playa."

"I hope you're right, James" I said and we went on talking about my birthday.

After I hung up with James, I thought about Tiffany for a while. I thought how could she have had anything? I didn't see any sores on her body, and she didn't have a bad cough or anything. Nothing like that, so I figured I was safe. I went on as I usually did on Saturdays.

That night my girlfriend called and told me she had dinner plans for us at the Choo-Choo. After we finished dinner, she also had a perfect night planned for us. Vanessa has been my girlfriend for three years, but she had a complex about shacking up together because we weren't married. I didn't complain about that because it gave me freedom and I loved that.

Vanessa was a high yellow, 19-year-old with a 5'3" frame and a very petite body. She was in her second year of college and majoring in chemistry. She kept me up on my responsibilities of being a man. I cared for Vanessa a lot, but I didn't love her like she loved me. I was still planning to marrying her with the hopes of my love for her growing.

At around seven Vanessa picked me up and we went out for dinner. After dinner, we came back to my place and Vanessa dressed up like a freak in her leather cat suit, stilettos, whips, and handcuffs. We always role played in our sex life. It made things more interesting. I loved it as well, but the activities from the previous night plagued me.

I didn't use condoms with Vanessa anymore. She never required me to but out of guilt, I wanted to. I didn't want to take the chance of giving Vanessa anything. However, I knew she would question me if I pulled out a condom, so I took a chance. Vanessa and I made love that night and enjoyed each other. She took my mind off Tiffany and what we did the night before. Vanessa always had a way of making me relax and comforting me. That's one thing I loved about her. Vanessa stayed at my apartment until Monday morning. She went to school from my apartment and I went to work. Not once did I think about Tiffany again during the week. I resumed my normal life.

On the other side of town, Johnny Peak argued with his significant other about staying out all weekend.

"Richard, I'm tired of this nonsense that you're taking me through. I don't need this crap!" Johnny yelled as Richard walked through their apartment getting dressed.

"Look, Johnny, back up off me, ok? I've been at Luke's all weekend celebrating his birthday."

"That don't make it any better, Richard!" Johnny yelled out.

"Well, what would make it better, Johnny? If I told you that I didn't do anything with anybody or if I told you I made love to one of the strippers at Luke's party, Huh?" Richard asked.

"Richard, what will make this better is if you just told me the truth and stopped all of the lying."

"Well, Johnny, yes. I had sex with one of the strippers, if that makes you feel better. And yes, while we're on the subject, I don't think I want this kind of relationship anymore! I want to be with a woman, Johnny." Richard yelled out. The words he spoke crushed Johnny. Richard was Johnny's first gay relationship and he was in love.

Richard and Johnny met at a gay club five years ago and had been together ever since. Richard had multiple affairs since they've been together.

"So, how long have you been feeling like that, Richard?" Johnny asked.

"For a while now, Johnny. I've never been honest with you. I've always cheated during the relationship, Johnny."

"With who, Richard?"

"With other men and women. I've found someone else I want to be with. I'm sorry, Johnny. I won't be coming back tonight. It's over." Richard walked out not to be seen again until months later.

For days Johnny sat in his apartment mourning the loss of his partner. He'd never lived another life besides the one he had with Richard. Johnny was 23 years old and Richard was 30. Richard was dressed in drag at a gay club Johnny attended one night with some girlfriends. He had never been with another man before he met Richard and since Richard, he hadn't been with anyone else.

Many months passed and Johnny went through his hardship by himself. He had no one to turn to after telling his family about his gay relationship. They disowned him after his coming out and he had no relationship with anyone but the gay people that he met through Richard; and at this point he wanted nothing to do with any of them.

*****

Chapter 2

If a wise man contendeth with a foolish man, whether he rage or laugh, there is no rest. Proverbs 29:9

Many months and Vanessa and I continued to have our relationship. I started loving Vanessa a little more and was thinking about asking her to marry me. I was tired of living by myself and waking up alone. Plus, I was true to our relationship ever since my party. My kicking it with James was even slacking. I was tired of doing drugs. That's all James did night and day. That's what I'm thinking when the phone rings.

"Hello?"

"Yo, what's clapping, Vic?"

"Oh, nothing, James. What's up with you?"

"I'm on my way to play ball at the Y. Do you want to go?" James asked.

Vanessa had to study for exams all day and I didn't feel like staying in the house so I went. James picked me up in his new Lexus 400 and we went to the Y. I thought I was coming down with a cold because I had the sniffles, but I didn't know because I also had a cocaine habit. I thought they could be from the powder so I didn't pay it any mind.

While we were playing ball, I got short winded and almost passed out.

"Yo, Vic, are you ok, man?" James asked.

"Yeah, James, I just should sit down for a minute, man. Gone and keep playing. I'm going to sit down for a couple seconds."

On my way to sit down, everything went black and I hit the floor. The next thing I knew, I woke up at the hospital a couple hours later.

My mom and younger brother, Mike were sitting by the bed.

"Hey, Mama." I said as I looked over at her.

"Hey, Victor, baby. Are you ok?" she asked in her soft tone.

"Yeah, Mama. What happened?" I asked.

"You passed out while playing basketball, Victor." Mike said.

"What?"

"Yeah, Victor. The doctor said that you had an overdose."

"An overdose, Mike?" I asked like I didn't know what he was talking about.

"Yeah, Victor. They said an overdose on cocaine." Mike said in the blunt way he always spoke to people. "Damn, Victor! How did you let James talk you into doing that stuff?" Mike asked not caring about cursing in front of our mother. "I thought you were smarter than that, man. You're my big brother and I love you, Victor, but you're stupid if you let dumb James entice you to do coke."

"Naw, Mike, I ain't done nothing like that, playa, So chill, man."

"Well, Baby, the doctors told me they found cocaine in your system." Mama said. "And they're running more tests as well."

I couldn't look at my mom's face because of my shame.

13

"Victor, baby, do you want to talk to me?" she asked. "Baby, you can talk to me about anything."

I turned to my mother with tears running down my face.

"I'm sorry, Mama. I think I need some help, Mama because the coke has become a problem."

My mother looked at me with her big, round eyes and put her soft hands on my face. "Victor, our God can heal our problems, baby. Let's pray about it and tomorrow we'll go and try to find you some help, Baby." My Mom bowed her head and I closed my eyes as she started to pray. "O, God, have mercy upon us, O. God, according to thy lovingkindness, according to the multitude of thy tender mercies blot out our transgressions. Wash us thoroughly from our iniquity and cleanse us from our sins. Restore unto us the joy of thy salvation and uphold us with thy spirit. Deliver us from blood guiltiness, O, God, thou God of our salvation and our tongues shall sing aloud of thy righteousness. Psalms 51. In the name of our Lord and Savior, Jesus Christ, I call upon your name my Father. Amen."

After my Mom finished praying, the doctor came in and told me that I was free to leave and he would call me when the other tests came back from the lab. That night I stayed at my Mom's house. Mike and I talked about my problems. Even though Mike was only 19 years old, he was very mature for his age. He understood my problem. He acted more like the big brother than I did. I loved my Mom and brother and they felt the same way about me. We are a very tight knit family.

Johnny continued to club for many months after he and Richard broke it off. He and Richard only saw each other in the clubs. Richard continued to do his drag queen impersonations. Even though they were no longer together, Johnny still loved to see him perform. One night they sat and talked after one of Richards shows and they went home together. Even though Richard was with multiple partners during their separation, Johnny didn't care as long as he felt warmth and love from the man he loved so much.

When Johnny awoke the next morning, Richard was gone and once again, he was all alone; it was back to heartache. Johnny vowed from that day not to ever give himself to Richard again. He couldn't take the pain that Richard was causing him. Plus, there were too many diseases out there. For the next month or so, Johnny got over Richard and moved on with his life. He even started dating another guy named Melvin. Love was kindled once more.

*****

During the Christmas holiday, I got a call from my doctor's office and was asked if I could come in for some more tests. Since I didn't think anything of it, I didn't mind. So, that Monday I went to my doctor's office. They ran several more tests and I waited in the little room while they ran them. I waited about an hour before the doctor came into the room. I knew something was wrong by the look on his face.

"Mr. Wilson, I have some very bad news for you," Dr. Little said. "Would you like to call your Mother before I give you the news?" he asked.

"Naw, Dr. Little. I'm a grown man. Besides, it can't be that bad, can it?" I asked more worried about the information.

"Well, Mr. Wilson, there is no other way to tell you than to be straightforward."

"Ok, Doc. I'm ready."

"Well, Mr. Wilson, you have the HIV."

I heard him saying I was infected with the HIV virus, but after that everything started getting quiet and my body got numb. I couldn't believe what I was hearing.

"Mr. Wilson, are you ok?" Dr. Little asked.

"Yeah, Doc., I'm ok. I just need some time to think."

"Well, you can have all the time you need, Mr. Wilson. Would you like for me to call anyone for you?" he asked.

"No, sir, I'm ok," I said getting off the exam table and walking out of Dr. Little's office. I went nowhere in particular.

I rode around town thinking about my life and if I had given this disease to Vanessa. I couldn't believe I slipped up like this. My mind was going a million miles a minute. I knew who gave me this death sentence. The more I thought, the more I thought about killing her, but in all truthfulness, I was as fault just like she was. I kept riding around until I got tired and then I went to my Mom's house so that I could give her the news. I didn't want Dr. Little to call her and tell her about me out of concern for what I might do to myself.

I arrived at my Mom's house around six in the evening, just as she was preparing dinner. Mike was watching the news with our stepfather, Raymond. My mother and Raymond has been together since I was four years old. He was more like my father than my real dad. He has always taken care of Mike, my mom, and me. My mom never worked outside the house and it was cool because Raymond didn't want her to anyway. He liked taking care of us, especially my mom.

I walked in the house and waved hello to them and went to the kitchen where my mom was. My mom looked at me and saw the tears in my eyes.

"Victor, baby, what's wrong?" she asked me as the tears fell freely.

I just stood there crying and not saying a word.

"Baby, tell mama what's wrong," she said as she came closer, grabbed my hands and wiped the tears from my face.

"Mama, I'm sick..." is all I said softly to her not wanting Mike or Raymond to hear.

"What, Victor?" she asked.

"Mama, I'm sick." I said more clearly for her to hear me.

"Sick how, Victor?" she asked.

"Mama, I'm dying."

"What? I don't understand, Victor."

"Mama, Dr. Little said I have been infected with HIV."

My mom stood there and her eyes filled with tears as she slowly started to cry, while she grabbed me and hugged me tightly.

"Lord, I know this is your will, but please Lord, not my baby." She spoke softly as she continued to hug me.

I backed up from my mom and wiped the tears away from her eyes.

"I'm going to be ok, Mama."

"I know you are, Victor." She spoke even softer as she wiped at her face. We cried even more as we looked into each other's eyes. "Baby, have you told Vanessa yet?"

"No, Mama, not yet."

"Victor, do you think you could've given it to her?"

I cried even harder at the thought of giving it to Vanessa. "I don't know, Mama. More than likely, yes."

"Oh, my God!" she said. "Not these babies, my God, not these babies."

"Mama, stop crying," I said as Mike came into the kitchen wondering why me and Mama were crying.

"What's wrong, Mama?" Mike asked.

"Nothing, Mike, just go back in there until I get finished talking to your brother."

"Victor, why are you and Mama crying, man?"

"Nothing, Mike, it's ok."

"No, it's not! Now somebody tell me what's going on."

"You've got to tell him, Victor." Mama said.

"Ok, Mama, but let's tell Raymond too. I want to get this out all at one time."

"Ok, Victor."

Me, my mom, and Mike, walked into the living room and she cut the TV off.

"Hey, Pearl, what are you doing? The news is still on." Raymond asked.

"Well, Raymond, Victor has some news of his own to tell you and Mike."

He looked at me and saw the tears falling from my face. "Victor, son, what's wrong?" he asked now more concerned after seeing that I was crying.

"Well, Dad, and Mike, I'm sick." I said, but that wasn't enough for Mike.

"Sick, Victor? What do you mean by sick, Vic?" Mike asked.

"I'm dying, Mike."

"What! Stop playing, Vic." Mike said.

"I'm not playing, Mike. I was diagnosed with HIV today."

"What, son?" My Dad asked in disbelief.

"Yeah, Dad. Dr. Little said that I have HIV."

"Oh, son, no!" he said as he grabbed me and started hugging me and now he was crying too. "Lord, please have mercy on my son." He spoke out. "Son, it's going to be ok. I'm here for you, no matter what I've got to do! I'm going to make sure that you get the best care." He sat back down in his chair. For the first time ever, I saw and heard my Dad cry out loud as he put his head between his hands.

I looked at Mike and he ran up to his room, not saying a word to me. "Yo, Mike, talk to me bro." I said. He kept running up the stairs.

My dad looked at me and couldn't stop crying, but he managed to talk to me. "Son, you hold your head up. Ok? There's nothing to be ashamed about. We don't have to tell anyone about this." Then he went back to crying with my mother trying to comfort us.

We all held each other and cried. After a few minutes, I walked upstairs and knocked on Mike's door. He didn't answer, so I just went in. When I went in, he was holding a picture of him and me that we took on his 18th birthday. He was crying.

"I'm going to be ok, Mike. I'm not going to die anytime soon, lil bro." I said. He continued to cry.

Not crying out loud, but tears fell from his face as he looked at the picture. I went and sat beside him on his bed and he turned and hugged my neck.

"I love you, Vic! You're my big brother and I love you."

"I love you too, Mike." I said. We sat there and talked about old times, until Mom knocked on the door.

"Can I come in?" She asked.

"Yeah, Mama, I think he's ok now." I said.

"Well, Raymond wants both of you downstairs so we can pray for you, Victor. Now you two come on so we can call upon our Father for guidance."

We walked down the stairs and my dad had his Bible open.

"O, Lord," he said as we bowed our heads and held each other's hands. "Hear my prayer, O, Lord and let my cry come to thee. Hide not thy face from mine in the day when I am in trouble, incline thy ear unto me. In the day when I call, answer me speedily. Psalms 102. My Lord, my son has fallen upon some troublesome times and needs your grace and mercy bestowed upon him. Give him strength to make it through the storm, my Lord. Let your blessings rain upon him and our family as we go through the suffering. I know, Father that you giveth and you can taketh away. And I ask in your name, Father, that this illness be removed from him. And in the name of Jesus I command this. Amen."

We finished praying and I sat at their house for a while. At around eight I got up to leave, but my Mom didn't want me to go.

"Victor, where are you going, son?" she asked.

"Mom, I'm going home now."

"Victor, I don't think it's a good idea for you to be at home alone tonight, son."

"Mom, I'm ok. I have to tell Vanessa. I think it's only fair to her, that I tell her soon, so that she can get checked out."

My Mom didn't want to agree with me, but she did and I left. On my way out the door, I kissed her and she started to cry again. I wiped her face and walked off. My Mom stood in the door and cried as I pulled away from her.

I went home, called Vanessa and she came right over. When she got here, I was sitting in the living room crying. She sat down beside me.

"What's wrong, Victor?" she asked as she wiped the tears from my face.

"Baby, I have something to talk to you about."

"What is it, Victor?"

"Baby, what I'm about to tell you, I promise you I'm so, so sorry."

"What, Victor? Tell me!" she said more anxious to hear what I had to say.

"Vanessa, I went to the doctor today and I was told that I have HIV."

"What?! Victor, you better be playing!"

"No, Vanessa. I'm for real baby."

"How, Victor, from me? I haven't ever messed around on you."

"I know, Vanessa. It was me."

"What, Victor?" She asked as she stood up from the couch.

"Baby, I messed around with this girl on my 21st birthday that James introduced me to. That night I got so drunk, I brought her home and had sex with her."

"You didn't use a condom, Victor!" Vanessa said in disgust.

"Yes, baby, but it busted and I didn't know until I got up."

"Don't you baby me, Victor! You've probably taken my life away from me! Just because you were drunk and had a one night stand. I ain't hearing that, Victor." She said and that's when the tears started.

I expected Vanessa to walk out on me, but she didn't. She fell into my arms and cried until we fell asleep.

The next morning, Vanessa didn't say a word to me. She took a shower and got dressed.

"Come on, Victor." She said.

"Where are we going, Vanessa?" I asked.

"We're going to the health department. I'm going to get tested and you need to be retested. If you gave me this disease, I want you to be with me when they tell me."

I got dressed and we went to the health department. It took them a couple of hours to do the tests and give us the results. My results were read first.

"Mr. Wilson, your test came back positive for the HIV virus. Your test Ms. Jones, also came back positive."

The doctor that read the results to Vanessa and tried to comfort us by telling us about the disease. He told us about certain classes we could attend with other HIV patients for comfort. Vanessa took it well and declined to go to any classes. She didn't talk to me for a while, but when she did, she told me that I was going to marry her and that we were moving in together. I didn't try to fight with Vanessa about what she wanted. I was just happy that she stayed by my side.

On Christmas, Johnny and his new friend, Melvin went to the gay club to watch the drag shows. They sat and laughed as the drag queens performed their acts. Richard came to the stage and while getting ready to perform his act, he saw Johnny with his new friend. He was furious at seeing Johnny with another guy, but he pretended as if seeing his lover in the arms of someone else didn't bother him. He performed his act and afterwards he came to the table where Johnny and Melvin sat.

"Hello, Johnny. How have you been?" he asked.

"I'm doing well, Richard, and you?"

"I'm doing well, Johnny." He said coughing.

"Well, that's good."

"Yeah, Johnny. Who is this handsome thing accompanying you tonight?" Richard asked eyeing Melvin.

"Richard, pardon me for my rudeness. This is my friend, Melvin. Melvin, this is my ex, Richard."

Melvin stood up and shook Richard's hand, letting it be known that he was with Johnny. He was the new queen in the picture now. "How do you do, Richard?" Melvin asked.

"I'm doing well, Melvin. Well, Johnny, I just wanted to give you your Christmas present." Richard handed Johnny a small wrapped box. "Don't open it until you get home because I don't want anyone to see my generosity towards you. I only gave the rest of them cards for Christmas, but I got you something extra special." Richard turned and disappeared into the darkness of the club.

Johnny put the gift in his pocket and he and Melvin continued to enjoy the night together. Around three in the morning, they decided to go home. When Johnny got home, he went to hang his coat in the closet. He thought about the gift Richard gave him. He removed it from his coat and sat on the bed to open it. After he removed the Christmas wrapping, he opened the lid to the box and was puzzled at what he saw.

It looked like a casket, but Johnny wasn't for sure. He pulled the little thing out the box and it was indeed a casket. Johnny looked at it for a while, then he opened it and removed a piece of paper from inside of it. After opening the paper, Johnny screamed causing Melvin to run into the room.

"What's wrong, Johnny? Are you ok?" Melvin asked as he sat by Johnny's side on the bed.

Johnny couldn't say anything. He just handed Melvin the box and the paper. Melvin looked at the casket trying to figure out why this made Johnny scream like he did and why was he crying.

Melvin realized the little box was a casket, so he unrolled the piece of paper and it read: 'Welcome to the wonderful world of AIDS!' Melvin dropped the box, and the paper. He looked at Johnny. He tried to comfort Johnny, but he was hysterical. He went to get Johnny something to drink. After Johnny calmed down a bit, Melvin asked him if this was the gift Richard gave to him. He said yes. They called the police to report Richard, but they couldn't do anything yet. They had to wait until Johnny was tested and proved to be positive for either the HIV virus or AIDS. Until then Richard hadn't committed any offense against the law. Johnny was relieved that he hadn't had sex with Melvin and Melvin felt the same way. The next day, Johnny went alone to the health department to be tested. While he was gone, Melvin packed his bags and left Johnny's house. He wanted no parts of HIV or Johnny. He got as far away from Johnny as possible.

Johnny sat in the small room, waiting for his results to come back. When the doctor came into the room, he told Johnny that he tested positive for HIV, and he was close to full blown AIDS. He told Johnny about the same classes that he had talked about earlier with the young couple. Johnny took the information for the classes and left the clinic. After he reached home, he got the note off the TV Melvin left for him.

It said that he was gone and wasn't coming back. He wanted no part of AIDS or him, and Johnny just broke down even harder. He lost his lover and his life all in one day, and had no one to turn to. He sat down on the couch and called his mother.

"Hello?" The woman answered.

Johnny didn't say anything, he just held the phone.

"Hello?" The woman said again. "Johnny? Is this you?"

Still Johnny couldn't say a word. The lady heard the voice crying.

"Johnny, baby, if this is you, please tell me what's wrong, son."

"Mama," Johnny finally spoke into the phone.

"Oh, Johnny, baby, how are you doing?" she asked.

"Mama, I'm ok."

"Why are you crying, Johnny?"

"Mama, I'm dying, Mama."

"Baby, talk to me, please come over to the house, will you?"

"Ok, Mama."

Johnny hung up and drove to his parents' house. When Johnny pulled into the driveway, his father was sitting on the porch. As Johnny got out his car his father got up from the chair, went into the house and shut the door. Johnny got in his car and was about to back out of the driveway when he looked at the door and saw it open. His mother came out and stood on the porch. Johnny got out of the car and ran up to her. They hugged one another as they cried with each other. She grabbed Johnny by the hand and led him into the house.

Johnny's father sat in the chair, pretending to watch TV. Not wanting to acknowledge Johnny's presence.

"Hey, Randy, look who came to see us. It's Johnny." She said. Johnny's father never looked his way. Johnny and his father were close until Johnny told him about his sexuality. Since then they haven't spoken a word to each other. Johnny's mom led him into the kitchen and fixed him something to drink.

"Johnny, why did you call? I'm glad you did." She said.

"Mama, I'm sick." Johnny spoke.

"Johnny, what's wrong?"

"Mama, I went to the doctor today and I was diagnosed with the HIV virus."

"Oh, Johnny, baby, I'm so sorry, son. Is there anything I can do?" She asked while fixing them tea and trying to fight back the tears that were threatening to fall.

"Don't cry Mama. I'm ok."

"I know Johnny, you've always been a strong young man," she said as they begun to talk. Johnny felt much better having someone on his side and someone to talk to. After they finished talking and drinking their tea, Johnny left the house and his mother sat down to talk to his father.

"Well, what did he have to say now? Is he having a sex change?" His father asked gruffly.

"No, Randy," she said as tears rolled down her face. "Randy, your son, our son is dying."

"That's what God needs to do with all of the homosexuals. They deserve to burn in hell for what they're doing." He said.

"Randy! He's still our son. He doesn't deserve this from you. You're an old, selfish man, Randy."

"Yeah, whatever, Julie. You've read your Bible and what God says about homosexuals, so why should I feel any different about him?"

"He's your son, Randy. And I'm his mother. I won't turn my back on our only son when he needs us the most." She said gathering her tea cup and heading to the stairs.

"Well, you do whatever you want, Julie. But don't include me in it," he said as she walked upstairs.

She prayed to God for her only son. No matter what his father thought about him. She still loved him and that's all that mattered.□

Chapter 3

Deal bountiful with thy servant that I may live and keep thy word. Open thou mine eyes, that I may behold wondrous things out of the law. Psalms 119:17-18.

Many months after I was diagnosed with the HIV virus. Vanessa and I moved in with each other. She still attended school, while I continued to work. We only told our families about our illness. I haven't told James yet because I feel like it's his fault I have the disease, but we still kick it every now and then. Vanessa hates when I'm with James now and she has no problem in letting him know that.

There was a knock at the door. Vanessa got up from the couch to answer it.

"Who is it?"

"It's James, Vanessa."

She opened the door and turned around to go lay down on the couch.

"Hey, Victor, James is out here." She said.

"Well, hello to you too, Vanessa," James said as he came into the house and shut the door.

Vanessa looked at him and didn't say a word. She turned away and turned the TV up louder.

I hurried to put my shoes on and ran into the living room because I knew that a fight between Vanessa and James would break out soon and I didn't need that. I walked into the living room, gave James some dap and went over to the couch to kiss Vanessa. She turned her head, so I could only kiss her on the cheek.

"Damn, what's her problem, Vic?" James spoke and Vanessa responded.

"You're my problem! I don't like you and I don't know why Victor keeps hanging around with you!" She said leaving James speechless. "Victor, what time are you planning on being back?" she asked.

"I'll be back before two, baby" I said putting my coat and hat on.

"No later either, Victor."

"Ok, Vanessa, I love you."

"I love you too." She said.

James and I walked out of the door. Vanessa gave James a 'get the hell out and never come back' look. When we got in the car, James looked at me knowing he lost that fight with Vanessa.

"Vic, why did you let her move in with you? We used to kick it until she moved in with you. Why does she hate me so damned much?" James asked.

"I love her, James. I got tired of waking up alone, playa. I'll tell you another day why she hates you so much."

"I've never done a damned thing to her little, skinny ass, Vic."

"Watch your mouth, James, before you say something stupid." I said as we drove to the club.

"Damn! Ain't we on the defense about our girl?" James spoke.

"Naw, James, I ain't on the defense about my girl. I'm just not going to have you speak badly about my lady."

"Oh, I didn't know you claimed that title there, Vic. Let me check this. The last time I talked to you,

Vic, she was just a bootie call, but now she's your lady?"

"Yeah, James, things changed with Vanessa and me. I'm even thinking about marrying her."

"Damn! She's got my man whipped." James piped up.

"I ain't whipped. Let's get off my girl and me. Just drive so we can get to the club before it gets packed."

"Alright, playa, but don't let me see you sweating the honeys tonight. 'I'm thinking about marrying' playa." James said. We laughed and started talking about other things, that's when Tiffany's name popped up.

"Yo, I know what I meant to tell you, Vic."

"What's that, James?"

"Man, that broad Tiffany has AIDS!" James spoke out like he was giving me a news bulletin. I turned my head and looked out of the window trying to pretend as if something else had my attention.

"Yo, Vic, did you hear what I said, man?"

"Yeah, James, I heard you, playa."

"Well, they say she is in the hospital dying, man. They say she's down to 105 lbs. That stuff has eaten her up, man. They say she's infected about 60 playas with AIDS. Damn, I'm so glad you wore a rubber with her man. I'd be messed up if she would've gave that stuff to you knowing I'm that one that put you up on her. I couldn't take that, knowing that I messed up my best friend's life." James was talking and didn't see the tears building in my eyes. "Yo, Vic, are you ok?"

I turned to look at him and he saw it in my face.

"Hell naw, Vic! Tell me that it's not true, man." James yelled out as he pulled his car over. "Damn, Vic! Why you ain't tell me, man?"

"How, James? What was I supposed to say, man? Yo, James, thanks for hooking me up with that fine broad, Tiffany. Oh, and by the way, she gave me HIV and I gave it to my girl?"

James looked at me as tears filled his eyes and he was stuck in a trance.

"Naw, Vic, tell me you didn't give it to Vanessa."

"Yeah, James, I gave it to Vanessa. I told her about everything. Now you know why she hates you so badly."

"Vic, I'm sorry man. I'm truly and sorry. I wouldn't have introduced you to her if I knew."

"I know, James. I don't blame it all on you, man. I did what I did and I'm accepting the consequences."

James reached over and hugged me as he let go of his hurt and apologies. I felt him, but I was all cried out. I accepted my fate and I'm going to make the best out of it.

After our conversation, I didn't feel like going to the club so I had James take me back home. When we pulled up to the apartment, James tried to pull himself all the way together. He didn't want Vanessa to see that he was crying. James had a reputation on the street of being a heartless playa. He had to be that way because of the business that he dealt in. We walked back in the house and Vanessa was surprised to see me back so early.

"What happened, Victor? Did someone get killed in that hole in the wall before you got there?"

"No, Vanessa. I came back home to be with you," I said sitting on the couch, motioning for her sit up.

"What's he doing back here?" She asked looking at James with disdain. Before I could say a word, James walked near Vanessa, knelt and hugged her. Taking her by surprise and making her speechless.

"I'm so sorry, Vanessa. I really am sorry. I never meant for this to happen, li'l sis. Can you find it in your heart to forgive me?" James spoke crying and hugging her. His gesture made Vanessa cry.

She didn't say a word to James; she just hugged him back as the both cried.

"I forgive you, James." She said returning hug.

James got off his knees and looked over at me and said, "If I can do anything for either one of you, please, please, don't hesitate to ask. No! I tell you what! I'll pay for your entire wedding." James spoke with excitement. I knew that it was more out of guilt for what he thought he had did to me.

"You two set the date and I'll do the rest. I promise you that it'll be the best and biggest wedding that anyone has ever been to," James spoke. "Ok, Vic and Vanessa? Will you at least let me do that for you?" He asked.

"Yeah, James. We'll let you do that, man. But you don't have to." I said.

"But I want to, Vic. You're my best friend and the only person in this whole world I can truly say I love and trust. You're my brother, Vic. The brother I don't have, and the brother I have done wrong." He said starting to cry again as we all hugged each other.

I must say that I'm glad that I finally told James and my family because I was tired of crying. I didn't have any more tears left.

*****

Johnny was involved in the HIV program. He would tell other people how he caught HIV, how to prevent catching it, and comfort someone that has been infected. For a while, Johnny looked for Richard to show up at the meetings. He kept a .380 handgun with him in case he showed up. He was going to kill Richard for what did to him. He never saw Richard in attendance at any one of the meetings. He was kind of glad that he didn't.

Johnny was Vanessa's counselor on the side. She never told Victor about Johnny and she never told Johnny about Victor either. But in a way, Vanessa was counseling Johnny because he would talk to her about his relationships with Richard and his father. Over the past six months, they became the best of friends. Vanessa thought it was time for Victor finally to meet Johnny, although she knew how he felt about homosexual men. Vanessa invited Johnny over for dinner Saturday. She felt that if she could accept James, then Victor could accept Johnny.

Chapter 4

Love worketh no ill to his neighbor. Therefore, love is fulfilling of the law. Rm 13:10

Saturday morning Vanessa got up, fixed breakfast for me and brought it to me in bed.

"Wake up, baby," She said placing the breakfast tray on the bed as I sat up.

"Uh oh, what do you want? What have you done, Vanessa?" I asked.

"Now why would you think like that, baby? I just thought I would fix and serve my husband breakfast in bed. Now is there anything wrong with that?" she asked putting the glass of orange juice on the tray.

"No, there's nothing wrong with that, Vanessa. If hubby hasn't done or bought anything to deserve this, then it has to be something that wifey wants."

"Well, Vic, I invited a friend over for dinner tonight."

"What's wrong with that, Vanessa?"

"Well, it's a guy friend, Victor."

"What type of friend, Vanessa? I hope not a boyfriend, because I ain't that freaky, baby."

"No, Victor," She said laughing while hitting me upside the head.

"Baby, he's a friend I met at a meeting."

"What type of meeting did you attend, Vanessa?"

"I went to a couple of those HIV support meetings. He and I instantly clicked. He's a really cool guy."

"Damn, if he's cool enough to get me breakfast in bed, then you know he's always welcome in our home," I said. However, I should have known there was more to it.

"Well, Victor, did I mention that he's gay?" Vanessa spoke softly.

"No, you didn't mention that, baby."

"Well, I just did. Are you ok with that, Victor?" She asked.

"Why shouldn't I be, Vanessa? I'm not homophobic."

"Well, it's done, Victor. His name is Johnny and he'll be here at six this evening. Victor, he has HIV too, so we don't have to be ashamed of our illness."

"Ashamed, Vanessa? I'm not ashamed of my illness, baby."

"Well, why haven't you gone to any of those support meetings with me, Victor?"

"Because you said that you didn't want to go, Vanessa. Besides, I have you for support, baby."

"That's so sweet, Victor. I was only mad when I said that I didn't want to go to any of those meeting, but now, I think it'll help us if we went to the meetings. There are couples like us and it'll help us deal with it better."

"Ok, Vanessa. I'm cool with that." I said.

"See, that's why I love you so much, Victor Wilson." She said eating off the tray with me.

We finished breakfast and went shopping for food. Vanessa wanted to fix her favorite baked pork chops, mashed potatoes, and broccoli for dinner.

There was a knock at the door, and Vanessa told me to get it. I knew who it was and so did Vanessa.

That's why she wanted me to get the door. I answered the door and was taken by surprise on how Johnny looked. I was expecting a small-framed man, with a soft voice and an effeminate attitude, but I was wrong.

Johnny stood around six feet-two inches tall, weighing around 240 lbs. of solid muscle with a Barry White voice. He made my six foot, 195 lbs. frame look small, so I tried to buck my chest out a little more, stood on my toes and deepen my voice when I introduced myself to him. He noticed it and started laughing.

"Hello, I'm Johnny and you must be Victor." He said.

"How did you know that?" I asked.

"Well, Vanessa has told me so much about you and you fit the description very well."

"Oh yeah? What did she say about me?"

"I'll tell you if you invite me in."

"Oh! I'm so sorry! Please excuse my rudeness and lack of manners. By the way, I'm Victor" I said holding out my hand to shake.

"Yes, I know and once again, I'm Johnny" He said laughing while walking in.

"Please, have a seat, will you?"

"Thanks, Victor."

As he was about to sit, Vanessa came into the living room. "Hello, Johnny, I see you've met my future husband and the comedian." Vanessa said giving Johnny a hug and a peck on the cheek.

"Yes, Vanessa. He's just as you've told me about him. He's a very funny person, girl." He spoke in his gayness now.

"I'm not that funny!" I said trying to be sweet and funny. They laughed at me, causing Johnny to respond with a joke.

"I know you're not that funny, because I've never seen you at the gay club in drag. Now, that would be funny." he said. Vanessa laughed even harder as she came over to me and gave me a kiss.

"No, Johnny, I don't think he'd look too good in drag."

"Ok, ok, enough gayness for tonight. I'm ok with you, Johnny." I now spoke with common sense; not afraid of Johnny's sexuality.

"So, Victor, who's winning the game?" Johnny asked shocking me.

"You watch basketball, Johnny?" I asked and heard how stupid I sounded.

"Just because I'm gay, doesn't mean that I don't love sports."

"I know, Johnny. I apologize for that stupid remark."

"No problem, Victor. Who's winning?"

"You know my boys is handling their business."

"Who, Victor, L.A.?"

"You know it!"

"Naw, Victor, Chicago is going to come back on them and whip their tails."

"Naw, Johnny, you must be crazy! Ain't no way playa."

"Well, let's put $5 on it and we'll see who's crazy, Victor."

"Bet, Mr. Chicago!" I said. Johnny and I sat down and watched the game while Vanessa prepared dinner.

I forgot all about Johnny being gay as we watched the game. He was a cool playa and I liked him, but not like that.

Vanessa was finally finished fixing dinner. We all piled into the kitchen. Vanessa said grace.

"Our Father, thank you for this day you have given us. Thank you for bringing us together to enjoy this meal. I ask that you bless us as we continue this earth. Bless this food and others that don't have this day. Strengthen us and may grace be spread around this world. Amen." And we went on to eat dinner and share conversations with each other.

"So, Victor, why haven't you came to none of our meetings?" Johnny asked.

"Well, somebody didn't tell me that they wanted to go to any meetings."

"I'm sorry, Victor." Vanessa said in her sweet, don't be mad at me, baby voice.

"Well, there's another one coming up this Tuesday. You should come. I think you'll have a nice time."

"If my wifey wants to come, then we'll be there."

"We'll be there, Johnny." Vanessa spoke.

"So what all do you talk about at the meetings, Johnny?" I asked.

"Well, some of everything. Anything from relationships, how we contracted the disease, and how we're going to help others that encountered the virus."

"Oh, that's cool." I said.

"Victor, is there anything you would like to say to me or ask me?"

"Naw, naw Johnny. Why would you ask that?"

"Because Vanessa told me you are homophobic."

"Naw, I'm not. I just have my thing about gays."

"Why, Victor?"

"Because you never know who's the woman in the relationship and they always try to holler at me and I ain't gay. Yeah, Johnny, I do have something to ask you, since you opened the can."

Vanessa shook her head like she was saying no.

"Shoot, Victor. You can ask me anything."

"Anything, Johnny?"

"Yes, anything, Victor."

"Well, since you insist, how long have you been gay?" I asked.

"Well, I've been out of the closet for five years and I've only been with one man. I've known I was gay since I was eight years old."

"Are you the male or the female?"

"I'm the male of my relationships, Victor."

"So, you don't like women?"

"Yes, I like women, but only as friends. I don't want to be intimate with a woman. I'm only attracted to gay men. I'm not into heterosexual men either." Johnny said. That made me feel more comfortable

41

with him, knowing that he only liked gay men and I'm not near that.

"Now, is there anything else you would like to know, Victor?"

"Yes. How long have you been infected?"

"Not more than a year, Victor. My friend gave me HIV; however, he has full blown AIDS. I haven't seen him since he gave it to me."

"Oh, I'm sorry about that, Johnny."

"Don't be, Victor. I've learned to deal with it since I've attended the support classes."

"I guess Vanessa has already told you about us?"

"Yes, I already know what happened. I applaud Vanessa for her strength to stay committed to the relationship."

"Yeah, me to, Johnny. She's my world. I don't know what I would do without her."

"That's cute" Johnny said in a homosexual voice and we all busted out laughing.

We finished dinner and sat around in living room talking. Johnny was a very cool dude and got cooler the more we talked. He wanted to start a program for people to go around and tell others about our illness and I felt that. I was tired of hiding behind the curtains about my illness, so I agreed with Johnny. I told him I would help him get the program started and would volunteer to speak to others.

We finished talking around ten that night and Johnny said his goodbyes. After Johnny left, I helped Vanessa clean and put the dishes away.

"Thank you, Victor." Vanessa said.

"For what, baby?"

"For being nice to Johnny."

"Anything for you, Vanessa."

"Now what about some loving?"

"Only if it's freaky and just us."

"Go ahead, Victor. Get the gay jokes out on me now."

"Naw, baby, I love you. Johnny's cool, so no more gay jokes."

"I love you too, Victor."

"And I love you too, Vanessa." I said. We kissed each other, then we went to the bedroom for more.

Vanessa and I attended the meetings for the remainder of the year and I got more involved with them. I became the spokesman for heterosexual men. Johnny became the spokesman for homosexual men and women. Vanessa became the spokeswoman for heterosexual women. We worked well as a team and started more support groups around the city, on the outskirts of the city, and groups for teens.

I got so involved in the work that I was hired by the State to continue with my work. Even Vanessa and Johnny became full time employees with the State. For the first two years, we were doing very well with our work, then the virus started affecting Vanessa.

Chapter 5

*O Lord, rebuke me not in thine anger, neither chasten me
in hot displeasure. Have mercy upon me, O Lord heal me, for
my bones are vexed. My soul is also sore and vexed, but thou O
Lord, how long? Return O Lord, deliver my soul. O save me for
thy mercies sake. Psalms 6:1-4.*

In 1993, Johnny and I were headed to Atlanta,
Georgia for an AIDS convention. We left Vanessa at
home because of her low T-Cell count was low. I
missed her already. The convention was to inform us
about new medicines that were coming out to help
fight the virus as well as information on prevention.
It was the first convention Johnny and I attended out
of town together.

Even though I had the virus for more than three
years, I've never seen anyone get real ill or die from
it. I've always heard that it was a suffering death. I
hated Vanessa being sick. I knew the convention
would be showing us films on the virus as well as
photos of people that expired because of the virus.

I really didn't want to see the films, but they were
supposed to make our understanding a lot better.

We reached Atlanta around ten that morning.
We immediately checked into the hotel. The
convention was being held at the same hotel that we
were staying in. As soon as I got to my room, I called
Vanessa.

"Hello?"

"Hey, baby, how are you feeling?" I asked.

"Hey, Victor. I'm glad you called. I'm feeling a
little better. I just got the sniffles."

"I love you, Vanessa."

"I love you too, Victor. Tell Johnny to behave himself and that I don't want him flirting with you," she said laughing.

It was nice to hear her laugh. I didn't pay any mind to her comment.

"Vanessa, I'm going to shower so I can get ready for this evening. Johnny thinks it would be a good idea if we go early so we can mingle with the others."

"Ok, Victor. You behave yourself and tell Johnny I appreciate him and that I love him too."

"Ok, Vanessa. If you need anything, don't hesitate to call me, ok?"

"Yes, Victor, bye."

"Bye, baby."

I showered, got dressed and called Johnny.

"I'm on my way out of the door now, Victor," he said without giving me a chance to say a word. I walked out the door and Johnny was already there when I opened it.

"Did you talk to Vanessa?" He asked.

"Yeah, she said she appreciates you for coming and watching out for me and she loves you."

"Did she say how she was feeling?"

"Yeah, she said she's feeling much better. She still has some small sniffles."

"That's good. Are you ready?"

"I guess." I answered. We walked onto the elevator and went to the lobby where they were holding the convention.

When Johnny and I walked into the main room of the convention. I saw pictures of people laying in hospital beds in some messed up states of illness. After we rounded the corner, I saw a young lady, no older than 12 or 13 years old. I thought she was probably there with her parents, but then I saw her with about five more young women. They were all walking around looking at the pictures and pamphlets that were lying around the room. For some reason, I couldn't get my mind off that young lady. She was a very nice looking young lady and so were the other five.

As Johnny and I were walking around looking at the pictures and pamphlets, someone called for everyone to file into the other room to watch a short film. Johnny and I went in and sat in the chairs positioned in the middle of the room. The six young ladies came and sat in front of us. The film started as soon as they were seated. We all watched.

During the movie, I had to turn my head a couple of times because of the graphic details. Some of the people in the movie had sores all over their bodies and some were in even worse shape. It made me worry about me and Vanessa. About how we might die. I didn't want to see Vanessa suffer because of my stupid mistake. Johnny never blinked an eye during any part of the film, he was so into it.

After an hour, the film ended and a gentleman stood up in the front of the room and started speaking. He told us all about the increase in HIV and AIDS cases across the US. Not only in homosexual communities, but in heterosexual communities as well, and has started spreading to teenagers. There were now over 150,000 teens infected with the HIV virus and over 10,000 with full blown AIDS.

I couldn't believe the statistics the man read to us. He said that over ten people die each hour from complications from the AIDS virus and the numbers were growing daily. After he stopped speaking, he had everyone in the room to stand up and introduce themselves. He asked us to share if we were HIV or AIDS infected.

The gentleman on the front row stood up and started the introductions. His name was Mike, was 38 and infected for 10 years and he was feeling better by the day. I thought to myself, ten years, he looked good for his age and circumstances. If Vanessa and I eat healthy and exercise daily, according to the statistics we could live a long and prosperous life with each other.

After everyone in the front row did their introductions, it came to the young ladies in front of us. The first young lady stood up and started her introduction.

"Hello, my name is, Mary, I'm 15 years old and I've had HIV for a year."

The second one did the same. After the six young ladies finished their introductions, I couldn't believe that all of them were HIV positive, and the oldest one was only 17 years old. She had the virus for two years. None of them had the virus for that long. I was shocked at their ages and how they handled themselves. They were very mature for their ages, considering their circumstances.

After the meeting, I took the opportunity to talk to the young ladies so I could get more information about teen cases. This was information I could use when I got back home. One of the young ladies told me she caught the virus from her baby's daddy. She said she had her daughter while infected, but her daughter never caught it. I was going to look more into that because Vanessa and I talked about having a child.

One of the young ladies told me that she caught HIV from a fight she was in with another girl. She said that the girl cut her with a knife and they continued to fight. After it was all over, somehow the girl's blood got into the cut she received during the fight. But what I heard from the first young lady infuriated me.

Her name was Vicki. she said that her father raped her when she was 11 and infected her with the virus. I felt sorry for her because she was only 13 years old and didn't have anyone to comfort her. She was in a foster home. Her mom was a crack addict. I gave her our phone numbers and Vanessa's name. I told her to call us if she ever needed anyone to talk to or for help.

After the convention was over, Johnny and I went to one of Atlanta's Comfort Homes for HIV and AIDS patients. We talked to several people that were infected with HIV or AIDS. Everyone had different stories about how they were infected. Some of the information made me worry about Vanessa and myself, while some brought tears to my eyes. I saw babies with the virus, and no parents. Their parents had either died from the AIDS or were out doing their own thing. I left that place and returned to my room. I took a nap until about nine O'clock when Johnny called me.

"Hello?"

"Hey, Vic, do you feel like having some fun?" Johnny asked.

"Yeah, Johnny. After what I've seen today, I'm up for anything that'll make me laugh."

"Anything, Vic?" Johnny asked slyly.

"Yeah, Johnny, as long as it's not freaky."

"Well, I've got the place for us, so get dressed. I'll be over in a few minutes."

I showered and dressed in 30 minutes. Johnny was at my door as I was about to walk out.

"Come on, Vic. I don't want us to be late," he said we walking to the elevators. After we got in the car, I asked Johnny where were we going.

"Don't worry, Vic. I've got some friends down here that'll cheer us up."

"Ok, Johnny. Man, I'm trusting you with my life."

"I got you, Vic. Just sit back and relax, playa. I'm going to make sure that you have a lot of fun." He said.

I didn't say another word and sat back while Johnny drove through Atlanta's busy streets. About 20 minutes later, we pulled up to this club that had a big pink sign on the front of the building that said 'Meows'". I should've known from the name and who I was with that things were not right. This was going to be a little funny. And I mean literally funny.

"Come on, Vic, let's go!" Johnny said as he hurriedly got out of the car.

I got out and followed him. When we went through the front door, I saw a Tina Turner look alike on the stage and I instantly knew where I was.

"No, Johnny." I started to say, but Johnny grabbed me by the hand and pulled me right along with him until we reached a table where some guys sat.

Two of them were dressed in drag. One of them looked like Patti and the other one looked like Whitney Houston.

"Girls, this is my girlfriend's man, Victor. Victor, this is Raymond and Carlos he said pointing to the Patti and Whitney lookalikes. This is Demond, and Darrell." They all looked at me like I was fresh meat. It made me feel a bit uncomfortable. "Bitches, back up! He's not on the market. I thought I told you that. Now let's make Victor feel welcome and comfortable," Johnny spoke pulling two chairs out for us to sit and watch the show.

After the Tina Turner lookalike got off stage, the spot light shined on us. That really made me uncomfortable. The Whitney Houston look alike stood up and started singing 'You're All I Need' by the real Whitney Houston. I must say, he sounded pretty good. Johnny got us a couple of drinks and that calmed me down.

After the fourth drink and the third performance, I was feeling good and enjoying myself. I laughed at the gay guys on how they were acting and the things they would say. I thought about Vanessa and wished she could've been with us. I think she would have really enjoyed the show.

Around two in the morning, Johnny and I decided to get back to our rooms. I told the guys I hoped to see them again and we left. Johnny and I talked about things on our way to the hotel. Johnny was now my brother and a cool friend. After we got to the hotel, I went to my room and saw that I had a message on my phone. It was Vanessa, she had called around one in morning, I called her back, she was still up waiting for my call. She said she just called to see how I had enjoyed the convention. I told her about it and the young girl I gave our number to. I also told her about Johnny taking me to the gay club.

Vanessa laughed at the thought of me being in a gay club. We both laughed after I told her about Johnny and his friends. Vanessa and I talked for a little while longer then hung up. I enjoyed and loved Vanessa so much now and she felt the same.

I went to sleep after our conversation and promised to see her the first thing in the morning.

Chapter 6

In May of 1993, I decided I was ready to pop the question to Vanessa. We were at my mother's church. I was singing a solo that day. After I finished the song 'Precious Lord'", I walked out of the pulpit and over to Vanessa.

"Vanessa Jones," I said taking her hand bending down on one knee. "You have been my friend, my love, and my life. I won't and don't want to go another day without you. Vanessa, will you marry me?" I asked. As Vanessa looked at me the church got even quieter waiting for her response.

"Yes, Victor," she answered. We held each other as Pastor Williams started to speak.

Vanessa and I went to her parent's house after church and told them the good news. They were excited for us and welcomed me into their family. I was happy. I was the happiest man in the world that day. I wished our lives could be that way forever.

We decided to get married on Christmas of the following year. Our honeymoon was in the Bahamas. We talked about having kids, but Vanessa didn't want to take the chance of passing the virus on to our baby. I told her about Vicki, the 13-year-old I met in Atlanta. I asked Vanessa how she felt about adopting a 13-year-old child.

At first, Vanessa was hesitant about adopting until I told her about the situation. She said she would have to think about it. The next morning, I called the adoption agency and told them about Vicki Wells. I asked them about the adoption procedures.

Even though Vanessa hadn't agreed with me on adopting, I thought I would at least get the ball rolling in case she said yes.

I gave the woman at the agency our contact information and told her about our circumstances, as well as Vicki's. The lady asked for my number and said she would get in touch with me after she checked on everything. I said ok and I hung up the phone and went to work. All that day I was hoping that the lady would call me back. I figured if Vanessa just saw the girl, she would fall in love with her. She was a beautiful, funny and lovable girl who needed some love and affection. We were the ones who could give it to her. Plus, she would bring the same thing we gave to her back to us.

The woman didn't call me back at work, so I left my office around six that evening and went home. I was hoping that she wouldn't call while I was on my way home because Vanessa was there and I didn't want her to know I had started the ball rolling until she gave me an answer. As I was walking in the door, the phone rang and I tried to get it before Vanessa did, but I was a little too slow. Vanessa answered the phone as I stood beside her. I knew it was the woman from the adoption agency by the way Vanessa was talking and looking at me.

"Yes, uh-huh, yes. We'll be at home tomorrow or we can come down there," Vanessa was saying to the woman.

After she finished talking, she hung up the phone and walked back into the kitchen without saying a word. I looked at her as she walked away from me. I laid my things on the couch and went into the kitchen where Vanessa was washing the dishes she had fixed our dinner in.

"So, are you going to tell me what she said?" I asked leaning against the kitchen counter.

"What who said, Victor?" she asked knowing exactly what I was talking about.

"The lady from the adoption agency, Vanessa."

"Oh, is that who that was, Victor? I thought that was the lady from the pet store down the street. I thought about us adopting a dog, since you wanted a child," She spoke.

"No, Vanessa, that wasn't a woman talking about adopting a dog. That was the woman from the adoption agency I called this morning and asked about adopting the young girl I told you about."

"So, you went on without me?" she asked.

"No, Vanessa, I asked the lady about the adoption process."

"Victor, you know you're really not a good liar and you never will be. But just to get this over with, the lady said that she could bring Vicki by the house tomorrow for an interview with us or we could come down to her office. We agreed that she could bring her by the house tomorrow evening around."

"Yes!" I said. "Vanessa, I love you! I know that you'll love her!" I said giving Vanessa a hug and a kiss before going upstairs to shower and get ready for dinner.

The next day, I couldn't wait for the hours to pass as I worked. I was so anxious at the thought of seeing Vicki again and for Vanessa to meet her. Time was moving so slow. At 5:30, I packed up my things and left the office. On my way home, I called Vanessa and asked if the lady had called. She said no and told me to stop by the store to get some juice. I stopped at the store and hit the expressway so I could get home quicker, but that was a big, big mistake.

There was a bad wreck on the highway that had traffic was backed up for miles. I knew I was going to be in traffic for a long time and that I would be late for the meeting. I called Vanessa and told her about the wreck and asked if she would ask the woman to give me a little more time. I didn't want to miss the meeting. It took almost two hours for the traffic to move and another half hour for me to get home.

Once I was on my way, I called and Vanessa told me the lady came and that she talked to Vicki and the lady left. I was upset about missing the meeting and not being able to see Vicki again, but Vanessa met her so I knew that would think hard about adopting her. I reached the house and I went in. I laid my things down on the couch as I usually did.

"Hey, Vanessa." I called her name and got no answer so I walked into the kitchen, but she wasn't there. I turned and walked back into the living room and up the steps to our bedroom. I heard Vanessa talking to someone, but I thought she was on the phone with one of her girlfriends. I walked through our bedroom door and got a big shock. Vanessa was on the bed with Vicki. They were eating popcorn.

"Why, hello" I said walking into the room with a big smile on my face.

"Hello, honey, I'm glad you made it home." Vanessa said.

"Hello, Mr. Wilson, how are you doing?" Vicki spoke with her soft and sweet voice.

"I'm doing well, Vicki. And you?" I asked.

"I'm doing good. I like Ms. Jones very, very much. She's so funny."

"I'm glad you like her, Vicki. But she sometimes turns into this mean old monster, so watch out." I said laughing.

"Victor, don't tell her anything like that!" Vanessa said throwing a pillow at me. "Vicki, I'm nothing like that, baby."

"I know, Ms. Jones. You seem to be a very good person and I like you."

"And I like you, too." Vanessa said.

"So, it's final? We're adopting, Vicki?" I said as I sat down on the bed beside Vanessa.

"Not yet, Victor. Ms. Richards told us to enjoy the week and weekend with her and she'll be back to get her Sunday night."

"Don't worry, Vicki. We've got you." I said. "That's if you want to stay with us and be our daughter."

"Yes, sir, Mr. Wilson, I would love that."

"Well, stop calling me and Vanessa Mr. Wilson and Ms. Jones. You can call us Victor and Vanessa, and hopefully later, mommy and daddy."

"I would like that Mr...." she started to say. "Victor" She said. We sat together and watched the rest of the movie. After the movie, Vanessa took Vicki to what will be her bedroom and I went to shower. After I got in bed, Vanessa and I talked about Vicki.

"I like her, Victor." Vanessa said.

"Enough to adopt her, Vanessa?"

"Yes, Victor. Enough to adopt her. I think she's what we need in our life."

"I know, Vanessa." I said pulling her closer to me. She put her head on my chest and I stroked her hair until she fell asleep on my chest.

The rest of the week I sat in my office, a nervous wreck. I was answering the phone on every first ring. I thought Ms. Richards would be calling me in the first couple of days of the week, but she didn't. On Friday around noon, my phone rang. I answered, not anticipating that Ms. Richards would call.

"Hello?"

"Hello, Mr. Wilson, this is Ms. Richards from the adoption agency."

"Oh, hello Ms. Richards, how are you doing?"

"I'm doing well, Mr. Wilson. And yourself?" she asked.

"I'm doing great. I've been waiting for your call this week."

"Yes, I meant to call, but I've been trying to close your case."

"Well, how's it going, Ms. Richards?" I asked.

"It's going well, but we have one problem."

"And what's that?"

"The agency is requiring that you and Ms. Jones be married before they give you full adoption of Vicki."

"Well, that won't be a problem. We're planning on getting married on December 25 of next year. Is that too late, Ms. Richards?"

"No, Mr. Wilson, but like I said, the agency won't consider full adoption until you and Ms. Jones are legally married. They are willing to let you two be foster parents until you are married."

"What does that mean, Ms. Richards?"

"Well, Mr. Wilson, it means that Vicki can come and live with you and Ms. Jones. And you two will be her guardians until you get married and then you will become her legal parents. Is that an option that you and Ms. Jones will consider?" Ms. Richards asked.

"I don't really care if we're going to be Vicki's guardians, because it would only be for a short time anyway, then we would be her parents. If Vicki is living with us, we could live as a family and give her the love and affection she needs." I agreed with the agency's conditions. "Yes, Ms. Richards, we would love to be her foster parents until everything else comes together."

"When will she be able to come and live with us?" I asked.

"Well, I don't know why she can't come today. She is here with me now. I can drop her off by your house this evening when you get home."

"No, Ms. Richards, I'm leaving work right now. I could come by and get her myself. I would like to surprise Vanessa with Vicki and give her the good news.

"Mr. Wilson, I'm at my office. we'll be waiting for you."

"Ok, Ms. Richards. I'm on my way right now." I hung up the phone, packed up my things and left the office.

I left the office right after lunch and went by Ms. Richards's office. When I got there, Vicki was sitting on the couch, combing her doll's hair. I walked over to her and gave her a big kiss on the cheek.

"Are you ready to go home, Vicki?" I asked not expecting to hear the wonderful response she gave me.

"Yes, daddy, I'm ready to go home with you and mommy."

Now that brought tears of joy to my eyes. I signed the papers Ms. Richards had for the agency and we left.

When Vicki and I pulled into the driveway, I saw Vanessa's car., This was the perfect moment. Vicki and I walked into the house. Vanessa was in the kitchen so I told Vicki to stay in the living room while I went to talk to Vanessa.

I walked in the kitchen. Vanessa was putting some plates in the cabinet.

"Hello, Vanessa."

"Hey, Victor." She responded.

"Baby, has the agency called us yet?" I asked.

"Naw, Victor they haven't. That bothers me. I was anticipating a call from Ms. Richards this week. I really like Vicki and I was hoping to have her by next week."

"Well, she called me, Vanessa." I said calmly.

"Yeah, Victor?" She spoke with excitement. "What did she say?"

"Well, come with me." I led Vanessa to the living room by her hand.

When Vanessa saw Vicki sitting on the couch, she ran over to her and gave her a hug.

"I missed you, Vicki! I'm so glad you're back." Vanessa joyfully spoke.

"I missed you too, mommy I'm glad that I'm back too!" Vanessa let the tears flow. She was so happy to hear Vicki call her mommy. She was happy to be here with us.

"How long is she here for, Victor?" Vanessa asked.

"Vanessa, Ms. Richards said she could live with us until we get married. In the meantime, we are going to be her foster parents. When we marry next year, we will become her legal parents."

"But will she be living with us permanently, Victor?"

"Yes, Vanessa. She won't be going anywhere. She's at home, baby." I said. Vanessa folded her hands and said "Thank you God!" "Well, this calls for a shopping trip, don't you think so, Vicki?" Vanessa asked her making a smile come to her face.

"Yes, mommy." Vicki answered. "Are you going. daddy?"

"How could I miss it, Vicki? I wouldn't miss shopping with you for the world."

"Let me get my purse and we'll go." She went to get it and we went shopping.

Vanessa and Vicki went crazy with our credit cards. Vanessa was buying girly things to fix up Vicki's bedroom. She brought outfits to match for her and Vicki. We shopped until the mall closed. I was glad the mall was closing, because I would have been bankrupt if they hadn't. Vanessa and Vicki spent over twelve hundred dollars and could've gone further. After we left the mall, we stopped by McDonald's to get something to eat. We ordered and headed home.

Vicki fell asleep before she could eat her meal. Vanessa smiled when she looked back at Vicki. She was happier about having Vicki than I was. I saw the joy in Vanessa's face that Vicki brought. We pulled into the driveway and Vanessa woke Vicki up.

"Vicki, baby, wake up."

Vicki opened her eyes. "Are we home, mommy?" she asked.

It made me feel good to hear that. Vanessa and I were parents now and we loved it. We said that we would take Vicki out tomorrow to meet our families. Me, Vanessa and Vicki, were so tired that we went in and went straight to bed.

Chapter 7

Shortly after we got Vicki, I set up a teen program for HIV infected teenagers. Vicki did most of the talking to teens. For some reason, teens listened to her better than us. I don't know if it was because she was a teenager or because she was an excellent speaker. But for whatever reason, they listened. I was just glad that they did listen.

It was finally the big day. I stood in a back room of the chapel, more nervous than a pig at breakfast time. This was the day I was marrying the woman I love more than life itself.

"Yo, Victor, are you going to be ok?" James asked while I leaned my face over the toilet.

"I think so James, as soon as I get through."

I was wrenching up my guts. It seemed each time I felt like I was ready, my stomach would turn some more.

"Dang, Vic, you're throwing up all your insides, man."

"I think I've been food poisoned, James."

"Food poison, Vic? Where did you eat this morning, man?"

"Vanessa cooked us breakfast this morning."

"Vic, stop tripping! Why would Vanessa want to poison you?"

"Maybe she don't want to get married, James." I wrenched some more."

"The way you sound, Vic, it's you who's afraid of getting married. Now hurry it up so we can get out there."

As James finished talking, I walked out of the bathroom stall wiping my face with the wet rag he gave me.

"Yeah, I'm ready now."

"Are you sure, Vic?"

"Yeah! Let's roll James." I said. We walked to the chapel where everybody was sitting and waiting for me and Vanessa. I walked to the front of the church with James by my side. Minutes later, the organ started playing.

The back doors opened and Vanessa's bridal party started walking in. They were all dressed in violet. After the bridal party was settled in place, the organ switched to the traditional bridal marching song Vicki came in with a basket of flowers. She walked down the aisle sprinkling them on the floor. Vanessa and her father stood in the doorway. It was the most glamorous and beautiful sight I'd ever seen.

Vanessa and Mr. Jones walked down the aisle. Vanessa's white dress hung on her body as does the wings on an angel. I watched her glide towards me as if she was moving on air. I was the proudest man on the face of this earth. After Vanessa reached me, I held my arm out for her. Together we turned to face the preacher as he started the ceremony.

Vanessa and I said our vows and then we kissed each other. I married the woman I truly loved. I was now a father and a hubby. I never felt any better. After the wedding and reception, Vanessa and I flew to the Bahamas where we enjoyed ourselves for two weeks.

After we returned from our honeymoon, Vanessa and I went on with the adoption procedure for Vicki. The adoption of Vicki was finalized on February 2, 1996. The same year that tragedy would strike.

*****

We were sitting in the living room about to watch a movie, when the phone rang.

"Hello?" I asked.

"Yes, is Mr. Victor Wilson home?" The lady's voice came through the phone.

"Yes, this is he."

"Mr. Wilson, this is Julie Peak, Johnny's mother."

"Yes, may I help you?" I asked.

"Mr. Wilson, there has been an accident. Johnny wanted me to call you."

"Is everything ok?"

"No, Johnny has taken very ill." She spoke only what she thought she should say leaving me to ask for more information.

"Well, is he ok?"

"I don't know. He told me to call you and tell you that he's in Memorial Hospital, room 218."

"Ok, I'll be right there." I said hanging up the phone.

"Baby, I have to go out for a moment. You and Vicki should watch the movie without me." I said getting off the couch.

"Is Johnny ok, Victor?" Vanessa asked.

"I guess. That was his mother on the phone and she didn't say much, except he was ill and wanted to see me. Other than that, she kept to herself."

"Victor, call me as soon as you know what's going on, will you?"

"Yes, Vanessa. I'm sorry, Vicki, baby. Daddy won't be able to watch the movie with you tonight, but I promise we'll watch another one tomorrow, ok?"

"Yes, daddy, I understand."

"I love you, baby. I'll call you as soon as I know what's going on."

"Ok, Victor, love you."

I kissed Vanessa and Vicki goodbye before leaving for the hospital.

When I reached the hospital, I went to the floor that Johnny's mother gave me. When I got off the elevator, I saw a woman standing in the hall. I walked to the room she gave me over the phone. The woman was standing outside the room.

"Hello, you must be Victor," she said holding her hand out to me.

"Yes, I am. You must be Johnny's mother."

"Yes. Johnny isn't doing well, Mr. Wilson."

"Please. Call me Victor. What is the doctor saying about him?" I asked.

She leaned closer to me and whispered, "Do you know about Johnny's sickness?"

"Yes, Mrs. Peak, we both work at the Care Center. Why?" I asked whispering.

"I think his illness has gotten worse."

"How long has he been like this?" I asked.

"He came to our house about three days ago with a high fever. I thought maybe it was a simple cold so I put him in bed and gave him some soup. The next day, I went in to check on him; he was sweating bad and couldn't talk. I called an ambulance. We got here yesterday evening and they've been running all kinds of tests on him since then."

"Did you tell the doctors that Johnny is HIV positive, Mrs. Peak?"

"No, I didn't. I didn't know if Johnny would want everyone to know that."

"Mrs. Peak, that's the only way they would be able to treat him. I have to tell the doctor."

"No, Victor. I think Johnny should be the one to tell them."

"Mrs. Peak, can Johnny talk?" I asked.

"No, but when he comes to, he could tell them."

"Mrs. Peak, Johnny could die if we don't tell them. We have to tell the doctor."

"If you say so, Mr. Wilson, but I won't have anything to do with it."

I walked into the room and saw the tubes running through Johnny's nose and mouth. The doctor was writing something on the chart.

"Hello, doctor..." I spoke looking for his last name on his ID badge.

"It's Ramsey, and you are?"

"Victor Wilson. I am Johnny's best friend."

"It's nice to meet you, Mr. Wilson."

"Please. Call me Victor. Dr. Ramsey, have you found out anything yet?" I asked.

"No, Victor. I had a lot of tests done, but most of them came out negative, so I ran a couple more."

"Dr. Ramsey, I might be able to help you out."

"I'm listening, Victor."

"Doc, my friend has been HIV positive over four years. That might be his problem."

Dr. Ramsey looked from me to Johnny. "He's so big." Dr. Ramsey said.

"Yes, Doc., because he eats right and works out a lot. Have you ever treated anyone with HIV?" I asked.

"No, Victor."

"Did you run an HIV test or a T-cell count on him?"

"No, because I didn't think he would be positive."

"He is. I believe that's what's wrong with him."

The doctor called a nurse in the room. She took more blood from Johnny while Mrs. Peak stood in the corner.

"Victor, I'm glad you informed me about his illness because the medication I was about to give him would probably have killed him instantly."

"No problem, Doc." I said as he walked out of the room leaving me and Mrs. Peak alone.

"I apologize, Victor."

"No reason to, Mrs. Peak. I know how you feel. You thought you were looking out for Johnny."

"Yes, because some people don't understand or want to treat a person with that illness," she said. By the way she spoke about HIV, I knew that Mrs. Peak wasn't comfortable with the disease. That she was uneducated about it.

"Mrs. Peak, HIV has been around for a long time. Johnny isn't ashamed about being infected with it. I don't know how educated you are on the virus, but it is nothing to be ashamed of. There are over 250 thousand people infected Americans and the numbers are growing."

"Johnny and I teach people every day about our illness. Don't be ashamed of it because your shame could have cost him his life today."

"I'm sorry, Victor."

"No need to be, Mrs. Peak. I think you should be better informed about this virus so you can know more about your son." I said. And as we talked, Dr. Ramsey walked back in the room.

"Mr. Wilson, I'm so glad you informed me about Mr. Peak's illness. If I hadn't known about it, he would have died by morning. His T-cell count is very low. I've ordered him some antibiotics. That should bring his T-cell count back up. However, I don't know how long he'll be in the hospital. I'm doing my best to get him back to his normal self."

"Thanks, Doc. I'm glad I could help." We shook hands and the doctor left the room.

I looked at Mrs. Peak. She was crying. "Are you going to be ok, Mrs. Peak?" I asked.

"I could've cost my son his life with my stupidity."

"No. Mrs. Peak. There are lots of people who think the same way you do. That's why we must educate them. People should know about the virus so they can help others live with it."

"I'm going to come to those classes, Victor. I promise. I really want to know more about it."

"Ok, Mrs. Peak. We have classes on Monday, Wednesday, and Friday at six in the evening."

"Ok, Victor. I'll be there."

"I'll be looking for you."

I sat there for another hour before I called Vanessa.

"Hello?"

"Hey, baby."

"Hey, Victor. How's Johnny doing?"

"He's ok for now. He's in a coma and they don't know how long he'll be in it."

"Was it from the virus?"

"Yes, Vanessa. His T-cell count was very low and it caused him to go into a coma" I said. This was a new stage of the virus for me.

"That's odd, Victor," Vanessa said."

"Why do you say that, Vanessa?"

"Because if Johnny has been taking his medication, then his T-cell count wouldn't go that low. Not low enough for him to go into a coma."

"What else would cause his T-cell count to get that low, Vanessa?" I asked.

"Well, it's one of two things that could cause that, Victor. One being, if Johnny stopped taking his medication and two being, if the illness has grown into AIDS."

"Do you think that, Vanessa?"

"I don't know. Ask his doctor and he might tell you. If he won't, then tell Mrs. Peak to get the information from him. If the disease has turned into AIDS, then he doesn't have much time left," Vanessa spoke. My heart dropped.

"About how long, Vanessa?" I asked.

"No less than 6 months, no more than a year, Victor," Vanessa said.

Mrs. Peak looked at me as I talked to Vanessa. I wasn't about to tell her what Vanessa was telling me. I didn't want her crying any more than she already was. I talked to Vanessa a little longer and we hung up. I sat there and talked to Mrs. Peak for a little longer and I kept looking at Johnny. I was praying that Johnny's illness hadn't developed further, but somehow I knew in my heart that Johnny's illness reached its peak.

After two more hours, I prayed with Mrs. Peak and I left for home. I thought about the film that Johnny and I watched in Atlanta. I hoped Johnny wouldn't go through that stage of illness and suffering. I also prayed for Vanessa, Vicki, and myself. I felt bad again about what my stupidity caused us. I rode home in complete silence.

Two days later, I received a call from Dr. Ramsey. He said that Johnny had come to and was asking for me. I left work and went to the hospital. When I walked into the room, Mrs. Peak was sitting in a chair watching TV and a nurse was checking Johnny's vitals. He gave me a big smile as I walked in the room and sat beside Mrs. Peak. When she finished, Johnny started talking to me.

"Hey there, Victor. I'm glad you could make it."

"Ah, Johnny, I wouldn't have missed coming to see you for the world. How are you feeling?"

"I'm feeling ok. I'm still a little light headed."

"Yeah, that'll wear off in time. What did Dr. Ramsey say?" I asked prepared to receive bad news.

"He said that he's gotten my T-cell count back up."

"That's some good news."

"Yeah, but he also said that the virus has turned into AIDS." I knew it was coming, so it didn't shock me much.

"I'm sorry to hear that, Johnny" I said trying to be strong for both of us.

"Yeah, but I'm ok with it, Victor. For some reason, I'm not shocked or scared. Going to Atlanta last year kind of prepared me for what was to come. I made myself right with God and now my soul is clear."

"That's good, Johnny. Vanessa said she's coming up later to see you."

"Yeah? Tell her she'd better make it up here and bring my niece with her. How are you two enjoying being parents?" Johnny asked.

"I love it. Vanessa is enjoying it more than I am. She and Vicki are always doing something together or buying something."

"How does Vicki like it?"

"I think she loves us just as we love her."

"That's good, Victor. I'm happy for you two."

"You need to hurry up and get out of here, so you can spend some time with her."

"Yeah, Victor, I know, man. I have something else to tell you."

"What's that, Johnny?"

"Victor, the doctor told me that I've only got about five months left, man."

"What!" I yelled.

I couldn't believe Johnny was telling me this. Vanessa was right. He wanted us to remain the same as we always had. I went with that. It made things easier. I applauded Johnny for the strength he showed me. I didn't know if I could be that strong, but Johnny let me know I could. We talked for a couple of hours before had to get back to work. I told Johnny I would be back later to see him and I left.

*****

Later that night, Vanessa and I sat in our bed and talked. I knew one day we would have to go through what Johnny was going through. Even though I hated talking about our death, I knew we had to talk about it and get everything in order. We had a daughter that we loved so much, and we had to make sure she would be taken care of if we passed on anytime soon.

Vanessa took out a $250,000 policy for all us. That made me feel better about things. I didn't worry about dying, but I wanted to die before

Vanessa. I don't think I could take living without her. If I did it would be because I had our daughter to look out for. Vanessa told me that she went to the hospital to see Johnny. She told me Vicki made them smile a lot. That it hurt her to see Johnny like that. That night, I think I went beyond loving Vanessa. I don't know what it's called when you care about someone more than loving them, but I did. That night, I held Vanessa tighter than I've ever done.

Chapter 8

Behold, the eye of the Lord is upon them that fear him,
upon them that hope in his mercy. To deliver their soul from
death and to keep them alive in famine. Psalms 33:18-19.

For the last three months, I watched the guy that I had come to love as a friend and brother die. I watched Johnny go from a healthy 240 pounds, to a mere 175 pounds. Not only did his physical condition change, but also his mental condition changed as well. Vanessa stopped in on Johnny at his house every evening when she got off from work.

Dr. Ramsey said that there wasn't anything else he could do for Johnny and there wasn't any reason to run up his hospital bills. He showed Johnny and his mother how to fill the needles and take Johnny's blood pressure. Mrs. Peak dedicated her life to doing that for her son for four hours a day. The rest of the day, a nurse would come by until 6 p.m. Vanessa and I would be there until 10 or 11 p.m. with him and another nurse stayed the night.

Vanessa, Vicki, and I dedicated our lives to helping Johnny and making him feel comfortable while still on this earth. There came a time in the last five months of Johnny's life, when Vanessa and I had to feed him and change his diapers. We didn't care about doing these things for Johnny because he was our friend, our brother, our loved one, and our strength.

In the fourth month, I stopped by one evening and met the man that gave Johnny his AIDS. I walked into Johnny's living room when the nurse informed me that Johnny had company. I walked to

Johnny's bedroom. There was Richard, leaning over Johnny's bed, holding his hand. Johnny smiled at me when I walked in the room. Richard raised up and looked at me.

"Richard, this is, Victor. Victor, this is, Richard, my ex."

Richard held his hand out to me for a greeting. Even though I didn't want to shake his hand, I did anyway. I was mad at Richard for abandoning Johnny after he infected him with the virus. Also, for the way he told him. It made me dislike Richard even more than I already did. I laid my coat and briefcase on the chair that I usually sat in, walked over and gave Johnny a kiss on the forehead.

"Richard, why are you here?" I asked not caring about hurting his feelings.

"Victor, not now, please," Johnny spoke to me.

"Naw, Johnny, I deserve this and if this makes Victor feel better, then let him get it off his chest," Richard said.

"I don't think you want me to get what's on my chest off because you'll be on a really bad end," I said to Richard. I wanted to take my fist and drive it straight through his pale face. His high yellow skin tone infuriated me.

"Victor, please! Not now, I'm happy Richard came by. Can you just be happy for me?"

"Yes, Johnny, I can do that for you. I'll deal with you later, Richard." I said, as Richard looked at me blankly knowing anything he said would get him hurt. "Richard, I apologize for my rudeness," I said.

"Johnny, I would like to apologize to you for what I did to you. I would also like to thank you, Victor, and your wife for being here with Johnny." Richard said.

"We didn't do this for you, Richard. We did this out of the love we have for Johnny."

"I understand your feelings toward me, but still, thank you." Richard said.

"you don't have to thank me. Hey Johnny, since you're doing better and you don't need me at this moment, I'm going to be leaving now so I can spend some time with Vanessa and Vicki. If you need me later, call me and I'll stop by, ok?"

"Ok, Victor. I love you."

"I love you too, Johnny," I said getting my stuff and walking out the room.

When I arrived home, Vicki and Vanessa had already set the DVD player up with a movie. I popped the popcorn, got us some drinks, and we lounged on the couch to watch the movie. After the movie, I told Vanessa about my run in with Richard. She told me that Richard has been there for the last two days when she went by.

"I think he has moved back in with Johnny, Victor. I'm glad he's there because Johnny needs someone besides that young nurse to be there at night with him." Vanessa said.

"Yeah, I guess you're right, Vanessa. But why didn't Johnny just tell us that he wanted Richard to stay with him?"

"Is he supposed to, Victor? Vanessa asked. "Baby, he's not our child. He doesn't have to tell us anything."

"But Vanessa, we're his friends. We're like family."

"But he is a grown man, and he knows what he wants. Baby, I know you've grown to love Johnny and you feel like he's our responsibility, but as for his private life - we don't need to interfere in it. Let's just be happy for Johnny, so when he does pass, he'll pass knowing we love him and he'll be with the man that he loves, ok, Victor?"

"Ok, Vanessa." I agreed.

"Now, why don't you come over here and give me what I need, boy? It's been two weeks and I've really missed getting it." she said.

*****

One of Johnny's nurses called while I was at work.

"Yes, Mr. Wilson. This is Nurse Maddox, Johnny's evening nurse."

"Yes, can I help you?"

"Yes. I'm at Johnny's house. I have been knocking on the door for the past 20 minutes and can't get anyone to answer."

"Ok, Ms. Maddox. I'm leaving my office now. I'll meet you at his house." I left my office and arrived at Johnny's house ten minutes later.

The nurse was still standing on Johnny's porch when I pulled up. I put my key in the lock and the door popped right open. I called out Johnny's name, but I didn't get an answer. I walked back to Johnny's bedroom. Upon pushing the door open I heard the thing that I regret hearing. I heard Johnny take his last breath. I felt a chill come over me.

I walked over to Johnny's body, felt it and it was still warm. I called for the nurse as I closed Johnny's eyes. The nurse came in and looked at Johnny, and then her watch.

"I'm putting 3:30 p.m. as his time of death," she said. She called for an ambulance to come and get Johnny's body.

I called Vanessa and gave her the bad news about Johnny. She cried as did I. After I hung up with Vanessa, I walked into the living room and sat down. I wiped my eyes and gathered my composure while I talked to the nurse.

"Mr. Wilson, where's Richard?"

"Excuse me?" I asked.

"Wasn't Richard supposed to be here with Mr. Peak?"

For the first time, I thought about Richard. He was supposed to be there. Where in the hell was he?

Twenty minutes later, the ambulance pulled up. The paramedics came in and started loading Johnny's body onto the stretcher. While they loaded up Johnny's body, Richard walked through the door. I didn't say a word to him. I walked right up to him and hit him in the face. Richard fell on the couch and I was right on him. I wailed on Richard for about 30 seconds before the paramedics got me off him.

Richard's face was bloody when I got off him. He never said a word to me, he just got up and walked over to the black bag that Johnny's body was in. He unzipped the bag and started crying while we watched.

"I'm sorry, Johnny. I'm so, so sorry, Johnny." He cried out until the paramedics walked over to him and helped him to a chair and began to work on his face.

"Victor, I only went to get him some chicken and to put some gas in the car. I haven't been gone for more than an hour. I promise," He said. He gave me the receipt from Kentucky Fried Chicken and the timestamp on it was 2:15 p.m.

I felt bad after I saw the time on it.

"I wouldn't have ever left the house if Johnny didn't want some chicken. I'm sorry, Victor." Richard cried. I walked to him and one of the paramedics grabbed me. I pushed him to the side and Richard stood up. We hugged each other and I apologized to him for what I did. We cried together for a while and the paramedics pushed Johnny's body out to the ambulance and took him away. I left soon after that, leaving Richard in the house to mourn over the lover he gave AIDS to killed.

I stopped at the liquor store on my way home and bought me a pint of Remy. I didn't by a cup of ice to put the liquor in, I drank straight from the bottle. I finished the whole bottle by the time I reached home. I was drunk for the first time since my accident. When I walked through the door, Vanessa was sitting on the couch crying. I walked over to the couch and sat beside her. She gave me a hug and smelled the liquor on me.

"Baby, I know you're hurting from losing Johnny, but alcohol won't bring him back or stop the pain. The only thing that liquor will cause is sickness. I don't want to lose you, baby. Promise me that you won't drink liquor again," Vanessa said.

"Ok, Vanessa. I promise." I said. I went upstairs to shower, kissed Vicki goodnight, told her that I loved her, then went to bed.

*****

The following Thursday, Vanessa and I attended Johnny's funeral. It was packed with all types of people. Johnny knew a lot of people from all over the south. There were people from Alabama, Atlanta, and from the Care Center. His mom sat in the front of the funeral home with Johnny's sister and the rest of the family. His father wasn't there.

I looked at the casket that housed Johnny's body. He didn't look the same as when I first met him. At the time of his death, his skin was much darker and he only weighed 158 pounds. He didn't look nearly the same, but my love for him was the same, so the shell that housed his spirit didn't matter.

Vanessa and I watched the love being shown, the pastor spoke his sermon, the good-byes being expressed and everyone crying at the sound of the choir singing ''.

After an hour of sadness and the preacher preaching, it was time for us to say our good-byes to the friend God had brought us. I walked up to the casket, bent down and kissed Johnny goodbye. Richard was beside me. I heard him saying he was sorry. I guess in a way, Richard and Johnny were like Vanessa and me. I loved Vanessa, but because of my carelessness I infected her with the virus that would one day kill her, just as Richard did to Johnny.

I couldn't imagine the pain he was feeling at this moment. I was hurt from losing a friend, but he lost a lover and a friend. I walked over to where Vanessa was standing, talking to some girls that came from the Center. I greeted them before and telling Vanessa I was ready to go. We left the funeral home and went to pick up Vicki from my mom's house. My mom had fallen in love with Vicki and Vicki loved her granny.

Vicki was special to everyone that met her. She was our angel from God and our strength. We left mom's house and went for dinner. After dinner, we went home and talked about the good times we had with Johnny. Vanessa went to sleep in my arms. I picked her up, took her upstairs and laid her in our bed. I loved tucking her in at night. It made me feel as if I was securing her a safe spot in my heart for the rest of my life.

I didn't go to bed with Vanessa. I went back down stairs to watch a little TV. I couldn't sleep. I thought about hearing Johnny taking his last breath and leaving his body. I always heard that when a person dies, the room will get cold for a moment. I heard it meant the person's spirit was leaving their body. I don't know if that was true or not. That's what the old folks say.

I stayed up until 12 or 1 a.m., and ended up falling asleep on the couch. I had the craziest dream I've ever had in my life. I was walking down some railroad tracks and this young girl about eight or nine years old was leading me by my hand into a train tunnel. I didn't want to go into the tunnel because I was afraid a train might come. The girl kept pulling me saying it was ok to go inside the tunnel. I followed her inside and I noticed a baby in her arms.

I didn't ask why she had a baby, but I kept looking at it and it didn't look real. After about 100 yards in, I saw a great big light coming toward us. There wasn't any room to step to the side and it was too far for us to try and run back. For a couple seconds, we stood there as the light got closer and closer. I was about to take off running towards the entrance when she pulled me by my hand and into a little crack that had a cave on the other side of it.

I looked around the cave as we stood on a narrow clay pathway. On both sides of the path there was nothing but complete darkness. It was like we stood in a bottomless pit. She pulled my hand again so I followed as she led. We walked for a while on the curvy path. Finally, we reached the end. That's when we walked onto a big platform and the pathway crumbled and fell apart, dropping into the bottomless pit.

I looked around the platform and saw nothing but bodies lying near the edge of the platform, suspended in mid-air. I walked to the edge of the platform to see if I could tell what was holding the bodies in mid-air. When I got closer to the edge, I realized that the bodies were dead people. They were lying on their backs as if they were laying in caskets. I moved away from the edge.

What I saw next scared me. One of the bodies I saw suspended in mid-air was Johnny's. He was lying there just as I saw him in his casket. His arms were folded, head up, and eyes closed. I bent down to get a closer look and that's when his eyes opened and he reached out and touched me. I jumped back so fast, I fell on my back. He went right back as he was.

I looked at the young girl to ask her where we were. She pulled me by my hand and helped me to my feet. She led to a wooden cross at the front of the round podium. After we reached the cross, I stood in front of it and looked up. The cross stood about 14 feet high and about 10 feet wide. The little girl backed away from the cross, leaving me standing there by alone.

A force I couldn't see pulled me up. A voice came out from above the cross and spoke to me as I dangled in the air. "Your faith will get you through this," the voice said. "You must not lose your faith. You must keep believing." I couldn't say a word, as I hung there in the air. Then a hand came out of the total darkness. It grabbed the gold necklace with the gold cross on it from my neck and went back into the darkness.

After that, I fell from the air and landed on my knees in front of the cross with my face towards the ground. After I stood up, I looked at my hands. I had the necklace in my left hand and the cross in my right. I looked in front of me and the cross was gone. Looking behind me, I saw the young girl reaching her hand out for me.

I took her hand as she led me back to the narrow pathway. While walking the path, I realized all the people that lay in mid- air were dead and I was underground. I was looking at the buried dead. After we reached the end of the path, I saw the small crack we came through. I looked back and it was pitch black. I couldn't see a thing behind me so I went back through the crack I came through earlier.

When I went through the crack, I was standing on the side of the railroad tracks. The light was still coming toward us. I looked at the little girl and started pulling her by the hand toward the opening of the tunnel. The light got closer and closer to us. I knew we weren't going to make it out of the tunnel. When I turned around to see how close the light was to us, I saw a lot of people reaching for me. They grabbed me and started beating and stomping me. I laid on the train tracks covering my face as the people beat and stomped me.

I looked out and saw the little girl standing there watching the people stomp and beat me. I heard her say, "If you only believe and have faith, then they will stop." She said it, but her mouth never opened. Still, I heard her talking to me. I looked at my hand and saw the cross shining brightly. I squeezed it very tightly and said, "I believe and I have faith." Then the people started to back away. I got to my knees and held the cross out in front of me.

Their eyes were a glossy white with no pupils. I yelled out at the top of my lungs, "I believe and I have faith." The people that attacked me started to backed further away. They floated backwards like ghosts do in movies. I yelled even harder and louder, until the people disappeared back into the dark tunnel. I then turned, grabbed the young girl's hand and ran out of the tunnel.

I realized that the people who were beating and stomping me were dead people too. Not like the people in the cave I saw lying in the air. Those people were at peace, not like the people on the tracks. These other people looked evil and miserable. They were all on top of each other screaming. I recognized that as I ran down the train tracks I saw the dead at peace, kind of like God salvaged their souls and I saw the souls of the dead that weren't at peace and knew that satan had salvaged their souls. I knew Johnny was somehow telling me he was at peace with God. When I looked down at my hand the little girl was gone. I had her doll in my left hand and the cross still in my right.

I left the tracks and walked through some bushes and fell off a cliff. I was heading for some water, but before I hit it, I woke up and looked around the living room of my house. I jumped up from the couch and ran up the steps. I looked in on Vicki. She was still sleeping. I went to my bedroom. Vanessa was still laying in the bed, just as I had left her. I went to the bathroom and took a shower.

As I showered, I thought about the dream and wondered why I had it. I think it was Johnny's way of showing me he was at peace. I finished showering, then went and laid down beside Vanessa. As I got close to her, I heard her saying as she slept, "If you only believe and have faith." I raised up and looked over at Vanessa's eyes, she was still asleep. That shook me so badly, I immediately started praying. I fell asleep as I praying.

Chapter 9

For the next couple years, we carried on with our lives. together with Vanessa and Vicki. In 1997, Vanessa and I watched our baby girl walk across the stage. Vicki graduated from high school a straight A student. She received an academic scholarship to Harvard University. Vanessa worked with Vicki on her academics since she came to stay with us. For Vicki's graduation present, Vanessa and I bought her a new car. She loved it. Vanessa and Vicki spent most of the summer preparing Vicki for college, while I put in more time at the Center.

The new HIV and AIDS cases had grown by 250 thousand since 1993. In the three years since Johnny's death, the reported cases of the HIV epidemic tripled. This didn't include cases that weren't reported. There was an increase in teen and heterosexual cases. This wasn't a virus only gay people caught anymore. There was no regard of race, age, or sex. It infected any and everyone that it encountered.

*****

Friday night, I got dressed as Vanessa sat in the bedroom talking to me.

"Victor, what time do you think you'll be coming home tonight?"

"Around two O'clock, as always, Vanessa. Why?"

"No reason, I just wanted to know. Baby, can you promise me one thing?" Vanessa asked as she coughed.

"What's that, Vanessa?"

"That you won't drink more than four alcoholic drinks tonight, Victor."

"I'll do better than that, Vanessa. I'll only drink two, ok?"

"Ok, Victor."

I asked Vanessa to come with James and me, but she said she wasn't feeling good. Vanessa had gotten more sick this year than any other year since she gotten infected. I wondered why she was getting so much sicker than me.

I finished getting dressed and the phone rang. It was James. Vanessa answered the phone. Even though James paid for our wedding and honeymoon, Vanessa still didn't care too much for him. She dealt with him because he was my best friend.

"Hello?" She said.

"Hello, sis-in-law, is Victor ready?"

"Yes, he is." Vanessa said scrunching up her face.

"Can you tell him I'm outside?"

"Ok." She replied keeping her response short.

"Why, Vanessa?" I asked.

"Why what, Victor?"

"Why do you still hate James so much? He's a real cool person once you get to know him."

"That's what you say, but in my book, he ain't nothing but a low-down snake."

"Vanessa, you don't know him like that to be saying all of that."

"Yes I do, Victor Wilson. He's with a different woman every time he comes to our home and if he's doing that, then that lets me know that he ain't nothing! I hope you're not doing the same thing!"

"Vanessa, come on, you know that I ain't like that."

"Well, birds of a feather, flock together. And he's doing a lot of flying and flocking, Victor."

"Well, I'm ain't flocking nowhere but right here with you, my love" I said kissing her and easing her back onto the bed.

"Victor, you better stop or you won't be going anywhere tonight."

"Well, if that's what you want, then I'll stay right here, just like this." I spoke in my charming voice that Vanessa loved to hear.

"No, Victor, baby. I don't want you to stay. You can go, but please be home by wot." Vanessa used her little girly voice.

"Ok," I said kissing. Just as I was hitting the top of the stairs, James leaned on his horn.

"Tell him we don't blow horns around here, so he can stop blowing," she said with much attitude.

"Ok, baby, I'll see you at 2:00." I said running down the stairs and out the door.

"Damn, Victor! What took you so long? The gate keeper giving you instructions before you left?" James jokingly said.

"Don't start, James. I ain't in no mood to hear it."

"Ok, Victor, I'll stop ragging on your wife."

"Do that." I said. "Where are we going tonight?"

"Vic, those out east playas just opened their new spot on Brainerd Road. I thought we'd go check it out for a second. If it's not jumping, we'll go over to Tear Drops."

"Cool, I'm down with that," I told James as I saw him pulling out his powder bottle.

"Yo, Vic, do you want some of this great grade A sunshine? I just knocked it off a brick I got from my playas in Florida."

"Naw, James, I gave that stuff up playa. So should you."

"I Don't do it like that, Victor. Just because you don't, don't mean I ain't."

"I'm not saying you can't because I ain't, playa." I answered back in the same tone he gave me.

"Well, that's understood then, Victor!"

"It is, James!"

"Look, Vic, I apologize, man. I just got a lot on my mind."

"Me too, James. So, let's just go have some fun and get whatever is on our minds off it."

"I'm game for that, Victor." We rode to the club shooting small talk.

When we reached the club, I saw a couple friends I went to school with. I got out the car and hollered at this guy named Roland.

"What's up, Victor?" He asked. "I haven't seen you in a while, playa. Where you been?"

"I've been around, Roland. I got married and I work 24-7, man."

"You're looking good, Victor."

"So are you, Roland.' I said.

"Hey, Victor, you know Carlos has his girls stripping here tonight."

Carlos is James' friend and he's Tiffany's pimp. He was the local pimp, with about 16 to 20 women he used to do strip shows, birthday parties, and special dates. Just like the date that James got for me. I tried not to think so much about that as Roland and I talked. We hung out in the parking lot for a couple of minutes and then went inside the club.

The club was jam-packed and it wasn't even 11 O'clock yet. There were no seats open for James or me. We walked to the bar and sat down. I ordered a Remy on the rocks. I immediately remembered my promise to Vanessa. So, I had straight alcohol with no chaser. After James ordered his drink, we turned around in our chairs so we could watch the crowd.

After finishing my first drink, I turned and ordered another one. As I was ordering my drink, I looked in the mirrors behind the bar and got a real shock. I saw Carlos coming through the crowd with Tiffany by his side and about four or five more girls in tow. I turned around in my chair to make sure I was seeing right. Sure enough, it was her. She still looked the same as she did in 1991.

James caught the look on my face as I stared at her while she walked with Carlos to the VIP section.

"Forget it, playa. She ain't worth it."

"I thought you told me she was in the hospital, dying from AIDS, James."

"Yeah, Victor, that's what I heard, man. I guess it was a lie."

"Yeah, I guess so, James. Or she has an identical twin or something."

I swallowed my second drink and started to get off the stool. James grabbed me by my arm.

"Vic, man, let it go, playa."

"Let what go, James? That she gave me HIV or that I gave it to Vanessa, man? That broad changed my whole life, man. She needs know it." I said snatching my arm from James' grip. I walked to where she sat with Carlos and his crew. I walked to their seats and stopped when I got close to where Carlos sat.

"Yo, Victor, what's up, playa?" Carlos asked. "It's been a long time, man. Where you been hiding out?" Carlos asked while I stood staring at Tiffany. "Yo, Victor, you ok, man?" Carlos asked breaking me out of my trance.

"Yeah, I'm ok, Carlos. I have a problem with your girl, Tiffany. Is it ok if I speak with her for a second, Carlos?"

"Why sure, Vic." He called out her name and she looked over at us like she hadn't done a thing to me. Made me wonder if she even recognized me.

"Yeah, Carlos, what is it baby?" She asked.

"Hey, my man Victor needs to holler at you for a moment. Come see what he wants."

"Look, Victor, don't do anything stupid. You only have 10 minutes, playa." Carlos spoke with authority. "You know she's working tonight, Victor. Time is money."

", Carlos. I won't have her for no longer than 10 minutes, man. Thanks."

"No problem, Vic... 10 minutes."

Tiffany followed me to the back of the club, where the music wasn't as loud. I turned around and Tiffany and I stood face to face.

"So what's up, Tiffany?" I asked.

"Nothing. What's supposed to be up?" She asked.

"Do you even remember me, Tiffany?"

She looked at me for a minute. "Yeah, I remember you now, you're Victor. James' best friend. I spent the night with you on your 21st birthday, am I correct?" She asked.

"Yeah, you're right."

"So where have you been hiding, Victor?"

"I ain't been hiding nowhere!" I spoke with authority, getting madder and madder at her for not acknowledging what she did to me.

"Why the attitude, Victor?"

"Do you know what you did to me, Tiffany?"

"What?" she asked, as if she didn't know.

"Do you know what you did to me, Tiffany?" I asked again more agitated than before

"Hold up with the attitude, Victor. Now you can tell me what I did because I can't remember that far back." She said with an attitude.

"Tiffany, why? That's all I want to know."

"Why what, Victor?"

"Why did you give it to me?"

"Give you what?"

"HIV, Tiffany."

"Victor, you're messed up! I haven't given you any HIV! I'm clean, playa. I just had a test last week."

I was angered by the way she talked to me and for denying that she infected me with the virus that's not only killing me, but killing the woman I love more than life itself.

"Victor, you have the wrong girl," she said turning to walk away from me. I wasn't thinking right at this moment.

I grabbed Tiffany by the back of her neck and slammed her face into the wall. I slammed her into the wall about three or four times when I felt a blow to my face. I went tumbling backwards. When I looked up, Carlos was coming toward me and cursing about what I did to Tiffany. He kicked me twice in the face and then reached down and picked me up. Just as he was about to deliver a blow to my face, James grabbed him and pulled him away from me.

"Hold up, Carlos! You've already done what you needed to do, so back up!" James yelled at him.

"James, that nigga is trippin', playa. He came and asked me if he could talk to Tiffany for a minute and I let him because I knew you. But when he gets back here, he started beating her, playa. I don't know what's wrong with your boy, but you better talk to him because the next time, I'll kill him."

"Ok. Carlos. I got him."

"Playa, your girl gave me HIV!" I yelled out at Carlos stopping him in his tracks.

"Yo, Victor, be quiet, man" James told me. I wasn't trying to hear that.

"Yeah, Carlos, the night of my 21st birthday, the night she spent with me, she infected me with HIV," I said as the crowd that stood around us got even quieter as I yelled my business out to Carlos.

"What, Victor?" Carlos asked.

"Yeah, man, she gave me HIV, playa. That's why you haven't been seeing me. I'm running the CARE Center for infected HIV or AIDS patients."

"Yo, Victor, you must have the wrong girl, man. I just had her tested with all of my other girls and she tested negative."

"Naw, playa. She couldn't have, Carlos." I said wiping blood from my lips.

"Yes, sir, Vic. I've got the test results in my wallet," he said reaching into his back pocket for his wallet. He pulled the results out and handed them to me.

I knew how the test results papers looked. What Carlos handed me was indeed the test paper the Health Department gives to you. I read the paper and it revealed that Tiffany was tested for the HIV and AIDS virus. Her results were negative for both HIV and AIDS. I stared at the paper and couldn't believe what I had read. I handed the paper back to Carlos, apologized to him and Tiffany and then I walked out the club, confused.

How did I get HIV if she tested negative? She's the only woman I've ever cheated on Vanessa with. There had to be an explanation for all of this. I couldn't have HIV if Tiffany didn't have it, I thought to myself as I sat on James' car until he came out the club.

"Yo, Vic, you ready to leave?" he asked.

"Yeah, James, I just made a fool of myself. I've got a lot on my mind. I don't feel much like partying" I said. James took me home.

We didn't say a word to each other the entire way. After we reached my house, I told James that I'd get with him later.

When I opened the door, Vanessa was laying on the couch watching a movie.

"Oh, you're back early? What happened to your face, Victor?" she asked realizing the cuts on my lips.

"I got into a fight." I said.

"With who, Victor?" She asked.

"Do you remember when I told you about that girl on my 21st birthday?"

"Yeah, Victor, but what does she have to do with you fighting tonight? I thought James said she died a couple of years back of AIDS."

"Yeah, he did say that, but she's not dead, Vanessa. She doesn't have HIV or AIDS." I said.

"What, Victor?" Vanessa asked.

"Yes, Vanessa, she was in the club tonight. I went up to her and confronted her about infecting me. After a small argument, I lost it, baby. I grabbed her by the neck and slammed her face into the wall a few times. Her pimp, Carlos, whipped my behind for what I did to her."

"After James stopped him, I told him about her giving me HIV in front of the entire club."

"Oh, Victor, you didn't, baby. Did you?" Vanessa said.

"Yes, I did. Hell, everyone already knew about me, so why not expose her too. No telling how many people she has infected. At least that's what I thought, but I was wrong. After I finished telling Carlos and the whole club about her, he reached into his pocket and pulled out her test results from the Health Department."

"What did it say, Victor?"

"That she tested negative for HIV and AIDS."

"What?"

"Yeah, that's what I said."

"Well, you know sometimes these tests will show negative results if the virus is in remission." Vanessa spoke. "So don't get all upset and confused about that."

"Yeah, you're right. I just wanted to look her in the eyes and let her know what she had did to me."

"Yeah ok, Victor, but did it make you feel any better?"

"No, it just got the hell beat out of me." Vanessa and I laughed although it hurt my ribs.

"Victor, since you got the bad end of the stick tonight, sit here while I go get some rags to clean you up." she said. I sat there while Vanessa played doctor. After she finished, I took a shower and went to bed.

*****

The next morning, I got up early, got dressed and left the house. I was planning to stop by my doctor's office and get another test done. I was plagued all night that Tiffany's results were negative. I didn't tell Vanessa I was going to my doctor's office to have another test done. I arrived at his office around 8:45 a.m. He administered another test. I left his office and went to work. Dr. Little promised to call me later at work with the results. I was cool with that, but for some reason, I was nervous.

I was hard at work when my office phone rang around noon.

"Hello?"

"Mr. Wilson, this is Dr. Little. I've got your results back and it reads positive for HIV." he said. For some reason, I was hoping my results would come back as negative. That would explain why Tiffany's results were negative. After I got the results from Dr. Little, I hung up and started reading a pamphlet I got from Atlanta when Johnny and I went. It said several things could alter a person's test. It said that a person's test could read negative, but he or she could still be infected.

HIV or AIDS would sometimes go into remission just as cancer would do, but it will come back later. That's why the disease is so hard to fight. Some people are carriers and some are spreaders of the virus. A carrier could have the virus for many years and test negative, but could or could not pass it to someone. Now the person that's a spreader of the virus would test positive for the virus and infect others. He or she would stay sick more than the carrier would. His or her symptoms would vary from a cough to a cold, or the complete illness.

That's when I thought about Vanessa and myself. I could be the carrier who gave it to Vanessa and if Vanessa had sex with anyone else, she would be a spreader. Even though I studied the virus and counseled others, I still didn't know everything there was to know about it. This disease changed form so much. That's why I attended meetings and conventions. To learn more about this deadly virus. After reading the pamphlet, I put Tiffany out of my mind. I went on with my everyday routine and got back to my life.

*****

The summer passed by so quickly. Vicki was off to college. We sat around all that Saturday night and talked to Vicki. Vanessa gave her lectures on her do's and don'ts. I just sat there and listened. I couldn't believe our baby was in college. It seemed like just yesterday I saw her standing at the convention in Atlanta and now she's on her way to conquer the world.

Vicki grew up to be a beautiful, young lady. She was mature and smart. I liked that about her. She said she was going to major in chemical science, so she could find a cure for HIV or AIDS. Her virus was almost undetectable now. Vicki was on a new drug that came out and it worked well for her. Her T-cell count stayed high, she was never sick, and when they tested her for the virus, her results barely showed that she was infected. Besides, Vicki ate right and exercised daily. That alone kept her system strong.

Sunday morning, we went to church. I gave myself to the Lord. I was already saved, but I've never been baptized. I was going to stop drinking and partying. That afternoon after church, I was baptized and I vowed to stop my sinful ways. After that, we went to my mom's house for dinner and then we left. We went back to our house and I put Vicki's bags in the car. We kissed her, said our good-byes and Vicki left for college. I hated to see her leave. Vanessa cried as she pulled off.

For the next couple of months, Vanessa and I spent time together, either at church or at the Care Center. I didn't see much of James because I stopped doing the club scene. I felt good and so did Vanessa that is until 1999, during the Christmas holiday.

Chapter 10

On December 10, 1999, Vanessa and I had just finished talking to Vicki. She was in her second year of college and doing well on her own. She said she would be home for the holidays on the 16th of December. Vanessa wasn't doing too good for the last five or six days. She went upstairs and went to bed, while I watched another movie.

At around 10 O'clock, I cut the TV off and headed to bed. When I got into bed, it was soaking wet. I called out for Vanessa to get up, but she didn't respond. I shook her and that's when I saw that she was sweating profusely. I called our doctor and told him I was taking Vanessa to the hospital. He said he would meet us there.

After reaching the hospital, the nurses rushed Vanessa back, while I filled out the paper work. Just as I finished the paper work, Dr. Little came out to tell me about her condition.

"Mr. Wilson, Vanessa has pneumonia and it's very bad. I've put her on the strongest antibiotic I could. She's awake and asking for you. Don't forget, she's very ill and needs her rest. Make it as short as possible."

"Ok. Dr. Little." I said. I went back to see her. They had all types of machines connected to her.

I walked over to her and she grabbed my hand as I looked down at her beautiful face. Tears welled up in my eyes as I looked at her and she shook her head, telling me not to cry.

"I love you, Vanessa." I said leaning over the bed railing to kiss her. She told she loved me back, with the little breath she had. "It's going to be ok, Vanessa."

"I know, Victor."

"Baby, Dr. Little said you've caught pneumonia and it's bad, but you're going to be ok. He said that you need to rest, baby. So just lay here and get you some rest" I said. She nodded and shut her eyes.

I pulled a chair up to her bed and I sat there until I fell asleep. The next morning, Vanessa's and my parents all came to the hospital.

"Hello, Victor. How are you doing?" Mr. and Mrs. Jones spoke to me as they walked into the room.

I stood up and gave them both a hug. "I'm doing ok, mom and dad. How are you two doing?" I asked.

"We're doing well, Victor. Your parents are in the waiting room."

"Ok, Mr. Jones." I said leaving the room to go see them.

"Hey there, Victor. How are you, son?" My mom asked.

"I'm ok, mom."

"Son, why don't you go home and get you a shower, change your clothes, and get some sleep. You're looking kind of rough, son." My dad said.

"I can't, dad. I can't leave her side."

"I know, son. But you have to take care of yourself too."

"Yeah, you're right. I think I need to do that. I need to call Vicki and tell her about her mother." I said. I went in and told Vanessa I was going home. She said ok.

I kissed her and left.

When I got home, I called Vicki and told her about Vanessa being hospitalized. I told her that her mother was doing well and she'd be ok until she got home. Then I took a shower and slept until around 9 p.m. that evening. I got dressed and packed enough clothes for a couple days.

For the next couple days, I lived at the hospital. I went to work and came right back to the hospital. When Vicki came home that gave me a little break. I did my paper work, handled our bills, and went back to the hospital.

*****

On Christmas Eve, Vanessa's condition took a turn for the worse. She started sweating badly and her temperature went up. She told me about an envelope in her dresser drawer. She told me to get it out and read it only if she passed away, but not until then. I gave her my word. Minutes later, Vanessa went into a coma. The doctors came in to work on her, but their attempts were futile.

Early in the morning on December 25, 1999, my lover, my friend, and my wife lost the battle she fought so hard to defeat. I had infected her with - HIV. She passed away on a day for love and giving, but for me a day of loss. Vicki and I cried standing in her room watching the doctors unplug the machines.

I couldn't believe she was gone and all because of me. I gave my wife HIV and it took her away from me. Vicki and I left the hospital around 6:00 a.m.

I called the funeral home and arranged Vanessa's funeral. Vicki helped me pick out the casket and flowers. She did the whole funeral business by herself. I sat and mourned my loss. For the first time in years, I took a drink of Remy Martin. I sat on the couch on that Tuesday afternoon and took my first drink in two years.

I drank so much it was Thursday afternoon by the time I came to my senses. Vicki was wiping my face with a cold rag.

"Daddy, you're killing yourself. You've been on this couch and drank eight or nine bottles of liquor. You can't keep doing this to yourself. I know you miss mama, and so do I, but we still have each other to look out for. I'm still here, daddy, don't you still love me?" Vicki asked as the tears fell from her eyes. She cried at the sight of seeing me in a drunken stupor.

I reached my hand up to her face and gently wiped her tears away. "Yes, baby, daddy will always love you."

"Daddy, you've got to pull yourself together for me, ok?"

"Yes, baby, I know it." I answered.

"Mom's funeral is tomorrow. You need to get yourself a shower, a haircut, and a shave."

"Vicki, what day is it?" I asked.

"Daddy, it's Thursday. We bury mama tomorrow."

"Damn, Vicki. Baby, I'm sorry." I said softly as I tried sit up.

"It's ok, daddy. Get yourself up and together while I run to granny's house for a minute."

I went upstairs to shave and shower. I walked past the mirror and scared my damn self, I looked bad. It looked like I had aged 10 years over the last few days. I shaved and showered. The shower made me feel much better. I went into my room and found me something to put on. I got dressed then went down stairs and threw out all the empty Remy Martin bottles. I went to the kitchen and got the other five bottles I had hidden under the sink and threw them out too.

After I took out the trash, I came in and fixed something to eat. It had been almost three days since I ate. I was starving. By the time Vicki got back, I had cleaned up the whole house, shaved, showered, and dressed.

"I see you, daddy," she said walking through the front door seeing me on the couch eating. "Now that's my dad there! A go getter and very strong Black man."

"Ok, Vicki, enough." I said smiling as she kissed me on the cheek.

"You telling me that you didn't fix me anything, dad?" she asked as I pushed her one of the three ham, egg, and cheese sandwich's I made. She bit into the sandwich and looked at me.

"What, Vicki?" I asked.

"Daddy, this ham ain't done."

"Yes, it is, Vicki."

"No, it's not, daddy." she said taking the ham off the bread and holding it up for me to see. Sure enough, it wasn't done. We laughed at each other while Vicki held the sandwich in the air. I guess all the alcohol I consumed numbed my taste buds.

"Dad, give me those sandwiches. We're going out to eat." She said. She took the sandwiches and threw them into the garbage. And when she came back into the living room, she smiled at me.

"Now what, Vicki?" I asked.

"Nothing, daddy" she said smiling at me.

"Ok, Vicki, what is it?"

"Well, since you keep asking, those liquor bottles that you called yourself hiding under the sink..."

"Yes, Vicki. What about them?"

"I hope you threw them away."

"I did, why?"

"Because I found them and emptied them out and filled them back up with water." she said. We both laughed. "I only did it because I love you, daddy." She spoke in a voice that made me do anything for her, just like all little girls do to their dads.

"Thank you, Vicki. I love you, too," I said. We left the house to go out for dinner and see my parents.

When I first went out of the house, the snow and brightness of the day hurt my eyes. I felt like a vampire caught by the sun. The rest of the day, Vicki and I rode around visiting people. She knew what I needed to make me feel better, just like her mama did.

At around 10 p.m., Vicki and I came home. I went straight to my bedroom. I was tired and I wanted some rest. Vicki stayed down stairs with some of her friends and talked about college life. It took me a while to fall asleep. I tossed and turned and wished Vanessa were with me. About an hour passed and I finally fell asleep with Vanessa on my mind and in my heart.

Chapter 11

The next morning, I awoke more tired than I'd ever been. I heard Vicki down stairs rattling pans and smelled bacon frying. I got up, showered, and dressed in my shorts that I wear around the house and went down stairs.

"I'm glad you finally woke up. I was trying to be as quiet as I could."

"That's ok, Vicki. What time is it anyway?"

"It's 9:00. Your coffee is already made and in the microwave. It's fixed just the way you like it."

"Why thank you, Vicki."

"No problem, dad. It's my job to take care of you."

"Ok, Vicki, what is it? What do you want or what am I buying?" I laughed making fun of her for fixing me breakfast."

"Daddy, I'm shocked that you would think like that about me, but since you asked..." She started to laugh. "I'm just joking, daddy. Now sit down until I finish cooking us breakfast."

"That smells good, Vicki."

"I know dad, thanks. It won't be raw." She said smiling and making me laugh some more.

Vicki kept me laughing. Even when she was a young child, she knew how to make me laugh and feel better.

I got the paper and looked at the obituary. I saw the picture of Vanessa and a paragraph about her burial. Vicki must have known what I was looking at and she asked, "Do you like it, daddy? It was the best picture of mom I could find at the time."

"Yes, Vicki. You are so amazing, baby." I said.

"I really miss mom, too," she said. I saw the tears coming out of her eyes and rolling down her face as she cooked.

I got up and gave her a big hug and kissed her on the forehead.

"I know you do, Vicki. I miss her, too. We still got each other. Isn't that what you told me?"

"Yes, dad. I love you."

"I love you too. I like my meat browned and not burned," I said watching the bacon turn black on one side. That made Vicki laugh.

"Well, go sit back down so I won't burn it, daddy." I sat back down and cut the news clipping out of the paper.

Vicki and I finished eating breakfast and we went to get ready for the funeral. The funeral was starting at 11:00. It was already 10:00 when we finished eating. At 10:45, there was a knock at the door. Vicki answered it. Seconds later, she yelled up the stairs that it was the funeral home people coming to pick us up. I slid on my shoes and suit jacket and headed down the stairs. We left the house and within minutes arrived at our church. Everybody was already on the inside waiting for us.

It's true what they say about us Black people, we'll be late for our own funeral, I thought to myself as I walked to the front of the church to take my seat. Mine and Vanessa's parents were already seated on the front row as Vicki and I sat down. The preacher came the back and walked up to the pulpit. He gave his condolences to us before he started his speech. Two people from the funeral home opened Vanessa's casket.

I saw my wife laying there looking as if she was asleep, the tears started running down my face. Vicki took out a handkerchief from her purse and she wiped my face, as I continued to cry. The pastor continued to preach his sermon and afterwards, the choir sang. They sang my favorite song, 'O Precious Lord'. The tears rolled down my face as my heart ached even more. I rocked in place as the choir sang. I said my goodbyes to the only woman I ever truly loved in this world.

I stood up, walked over to Vanessa, I leaned over and kissed her lips and then I whispered, "I'll see you in heaven, baby. Save me a spot." After that, I went back to my seat. After I sat down, the congregation made its way to say their goodbyes.

After the funeral, we left the church and went over to my parents' home for the repast. Vicki and I sat around and ate talking with people that came over. There was so much food, I ate twice while we were there. After everyone left, I helped my mom and Vicki straighten up the house and then we left. Vicki dropped me off at home and said that she would be back after she dropped off a couple of her friends. I told her I was ok and to go on and have herself some fun. Besides, I needed some time alone.

I went in the house, undressed, and laid down on the bed. And for some reason, the letter that Vanessa told me about crossed my mind. I got up and went over to her dresser to get the envelope and sure enough, it was sitting right where she told me it would be. I got the envelope and sat back on the bed. I opened the letter and it read it.

Hello Victor,

I assume if you're reading this letter, then I've passed on. I'm sorry I'm not there for you, but I know Vicki is watching out for you. Victor, you were my world, my love and my life. I've never loved anyone as much as I've loved you. What I'm about to tell you I wish I could've told you while I was still there with you, but I couldn't and I hope that you can forgive me for what I'm about to say. Do you remember when you and I first met at the diner over on third street? I hope you do. That day when you walked in, I thought that you were the angel from heaven that God sent to me. See Victor, I decided that day, I was going to take my own life later that night. Victor, I was going through something I was keeping a secret for a long time. I couldn't hold it any longer. But before I tell you what my secret is, Victor, let me tell you the story behind it and why I hid it for so long.

When I came to Chattanooga to go to school back in 1989, I met some friends and they introduced me to this guy. I kicked it with him for about six months. I finally got tired of him, so I let him go and I went my way. One day, about six months after I broke up with that guy, my school was having a blood drive and I donated some of my blood. Well, two weeks later, I got a call from the Dean, telling me to come to his office and I went. When I got to his office, I saw the woman who took my blood at the blood drive. I was nervous, but I went in. After I sat down, the Dean left the lady and me alone. That's when she told me. Victor, I tested positive for HIV back in 1989. I was so hurt, that I brought a gun and looked for that guy for almost a year. I never found him. I was tired of looking for him the night I met you in that diner. I was tired of hiding the secret and tired of living with HIV, until I met you.

Before I tell you my secret Victor, please believe me when I tell you that I never meant to infect you with the HIV virus. That's why when we made love, I made you wear a condom. But after the one-year mark, you told me that you had a condom on, but you never put one on. That's why when you came into the bathroom and told me you never put the condom on, I started crying. You thought I was crying because I was scared that I would get pregnant. Victor, I was crying because I knew you were infected with the virus and I didn't have enough heart to tell you. Victor, I loved you and I didn't want to lose you, so I didn't say anything. Please forgive me, Victor. After what happened, I was still holding all the pain that I was holding inside. About two months after that, you invited some of your friends over to your apartment while I was over there with you. Victor, when your friends James, Raymond, and

William came through the door, I was shocked. I was looking face to face with the guy who infected me with the HIV virus. I was so mad at him. I wanted to reach in my pocket book, get my gun, and blow his damned brains out.

Baby, you've asked me so many times why I hated James so much. Victor, James is the one who infected me with HIV. When he saw me with you that night he got scared and thought I was going to tell you about him. I was scared that he was going to tell you about us and what he did to me.

That's when he came into the kitchen while I was fixing you something to eat.

He told me he wasn't going to tell you about us. I told him that he gave me the virus.

That's when he told me he was sorry, and that he knew that he was infected before we got together. He said that the condom busted and that's why he started treating me like he did. He said that he was glad that I broke up with him and that he would take care of you if I just kept my mouth closed about him being infected and giving it to me. That's why he hooked you up with that girl Tiffany on your 21st birthday. He thought she had the virus and he knew you would have sex with her that night.

The condoms that gave you that night were messed up. They were old and they were known to bust. Baby, I swear if I knew what he was doing then, I promise I would have told you everything. After you had sex with Tiffany that night, James knew the condom had busted on you. That morning he called me and told me all about what he had did to you. He knew you would think that Tiffany gave you the virus and you would think that you gave it to me. That way you wouldn't know that he and I messed around and that he was the one who infected me with the virus that took my life and that I've given to the only man that I've ever loved in my time on God's earth.

Victor, James has had the virus since 1987 and he's been spreading it ever since. I wish I could've told you this while I was still alive, but like I said, Victor, I feared you leaving me. I couldn't handle that. I didn't want to handle that. Victor, please forgive me, baby so my soul can be at peace and I can rest until I see you again.

Love,

Vanessa

The tears fell down my face as I finished reading the letter.

"I forgive you, Vanessa. I'll love you always," I said looking up at the ceiling trying to look into heaven at her. It hurt to know the woman I dedicated my life to, promised to love and honor, held this secret from me. Even though she held it from me, I wasn't mad at her and couldn't be, even if I wanted to. I folded the letter, put it in my drawer, and laid back down on the bed. I was looking up at the ceiling and thinking about Vanessa, when I felt the tears rolling.

"I forgive you, Vanessa. I pray you are at peace and with our Lord, baby, until I come." I said lying there until I fell asleep heart broken.

Chapter 12

Vicki and I celebrated New Years at church with my parents. After the service, Vicki took her new boyfriend, Aaron home. He knew about Vicki's illness. It didn't matter to him. Even though I didn't want to talk to my baby about sex and protection, I did anyway. One day when she first met Aaron. They both understood and they continued to date each other and have been together now for a month.

Later that night, I needed some air, so I rode around town. I was riding and letting my mind wander until I saw James going into a club on ninth street. I parked and went in. I walked up to the bar where James was sitting by himself. I sat on the stool beside him.

"Hello, James" I said. He looked as if he saw a ghost.

"What's up, Vic? How's life been treating you?"

"Well, James. You?"

"It's been fair, Victor. Vic, I'm sorry about Vanessa, man."

"Yeah, James. Thanks."

"What brings you out to the club scene tonight, Victor?" he asked. "I thought you were through with this life."

"I am, but I saw you coming in here and I had to talk to you."

"About what, Victor?"

"About Vanessa."

"What about her, Victor?"

"She told me, James."

"Told you what, Vic?"

"About you and her and that you infected her. How you played me with Tiffany and how you called her and told her your plan."

"Vic, what? You must be tripping or your bitch is." He said apparently, without thinking about what I was about to do to him for disrespecting her.

I drew back my fist and knocked James out of his chair and onto the floor.

"James, you could've said what you wanted to about me, but I'll be damned if I let you disrespect my wife!" I said. James got up off the floor and looked at me. "Victor, you don't have any proof about what she said, so fuck you!" He said. I just looked at him and walked out of the club and went home.

The next morning, I called Chief Dodson and told him what James was doing. Later that night, I saw James on the news in handcuffs, being taken into the County Jail. They were charging him with first degree murder of Vanessa and attempted murder of 50 other women. I smiled as I thought about Vanessa finally getting her revenge on James., I went upstairs and went to sleep.

While I was asleep, I had that dream again, but this time I saw Vanessa lying there and you know the rest. Vicki and I continued to live each day, loving one another and telling people about being aware of the HIV and AIDS viruses until 2002, when I became real ill.

I went to the hospital. My mom called Vicki and told her. Vicki came right down and right to the hospital. She only had a few more years before she would graduate with her Master' Degree.

She was sitting and talking to me while I was writing in my diary. "Dad, what's that you're writing in?" Vicki asked.

"Oh, it's a book that I've been writing about my life's battle with HIV, Vicki." After telling her about the book, I told her that I was going to take a nap because I was very tired.

*****

That night my father never awoke from the nap he took. My dad passed away peacefully in his sleep. My dad was born September 10, 1970 and passed in July of 2002. After I left the hospital, I went home and read this book. I cried as I read it and thought about my parents. I thanked God for them and the life they gave me. If it wasn't for them, I wouldn't have had the type of life I have. I wouldn't be who I am. Today and forever forward, I will dedicate my life to the cause they lived and died for. May God bless their souls and may they rest in peace.

That night I laid on their bed and fell asleep. I had the weirdest dream about my parents and Uncle Johnny. I was walking on these railroad tracks and this little girl was leading me into this tunnel by my hand. She had this doll in her hand and it looked real, but it wasn't. I followed the little girl and when we got inside of the tunnel, a bright light was coming toward us and she pulled me into a crack in the tunnel wall. Inside of this crack was a cave that was pitch black. I couldn't see a thing but the pathway I walked on.

The little girl led me on around this path to a podium. Once we got onto it, the pathway we walked on crumbled and fell into the darkness. I never heard it hit the bottom of the cave. I looked around and saw people floating in mid-air. I walked over to the edge to see the bodies. When I got there, it was my parents and Uncle Johnny I saw lying there in peace.

I bent down to get a better look and that's when my father's eyes opened and he sat up.

"Hello, Vicki." He said. "I hope that you are well. Your mother, Uncle Johnny, and I are doing well and will always be with you. Vicki, our deaths were for a good cause, as was our lives. Continue to do the work you're doing. We love you, Vicki" my father said. Then he laid back down.

After I stood up, I walked over to the little girl and she walked me back out into the tunnel. After we got to it, I saw the light coming toward us and I too ran toward the entrance. I never made it to the entrance because a hand grabbed me and I turned around. When I did, I saw James and he looked weird. His eyes were glassy white with no pupils. He looked as if he were in pain. He was screaming something, but I couldn't understand what he was saying. It scared me. I tried to break away from him, but couldn't until I held my hand up and realized I had this gold cross in my hand.

I don't know where the cross came from, but I had it in my hand. When I raised it up, James saw the cross and he started backing up like vampires do in the movies. Then I saw more people grabbing James as he went backwards screaming. I turned and ran out of the tunnel. After I got to the entrance, I woke up from my dream sweating so badly that I had to take a shower.

As I was going to the shower, I glanced at the TV and a reporter was saying something about a suicide at the County Jail. I sat on the bed and heard James' name being mentioned. They said that James Thomas was found hanging in his cell, dead from an apparent suicide. I couldn't believe what I was hearing. I thought about my dream. I looked at the ceiling and told my parents and Uncle Johnny that I loved them, then went to take my shower.

One year passed before I had to attend Richard's funeral. Richard started helping me with the Care Center and doing speaking engagements around the world about HIV and AIDS.

I am a medical scientist and had developed a new drug to fight off HIV. I was taking the drug myself. As of late, I've tested negative for the virus. I don't know how long it'll take before the drug will be approved by the FDA, but it should be soon.

I thank you for reading the story my dad died writing and I completed. I thank God for the souls that he has salvaged from the HIV and AIDS viruses. I pray that your understanding of this virus is enhanced.

THE END